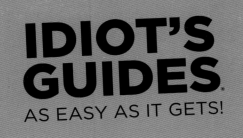

IDIOT'S GUIDES®
AS EASY AS IT GETS!

Everyday Makeup Secrets

D1473299

by Daniel Klingler

ALPHA

A member of Penguin Random House LLC

Published by Penguin Random House LLC

Penguin Random House LLC, 375 Hudson Street, New York, New York 10014, USA · Penguin Random House LLC (Canada), 90 Eglinton Avenue East, Suite 700, Toronto, Ontario M4P 2Y3, Canada (a division of Pearson Penguin Canada Inc.) · Penguin Books Ltd., 80 Strand, London WC2R 0RL, England · Penguin Ireland, 25 St. Stephen's Green, Dublin 2, Ireland (a division of Penguin Books Ltd.) · Penguin Random House LLC (Australia), 250 Camberwell Road, Camberwell, Victoria 3124, Australia (a division of Pearson Australia Group Pty. Ltd.) · Penguin Books India Pvt. Ltd., 11 Community Centre, Panchsheel Park, New Delhi—110 017, India · Penguin Random House LLC (NZ), 67 Apollo Drive, Rosedale, North Shore, Auckland 1311, New Zealand (a division of Pearson New Zealand Ltd.) · Penguin Books (South Africa) (Pty.) Ltd., 24 Sturdee Avenue, Rosebank, Johannesburg 2196, South Africa · Penguin Books Ltd., Registered Offices: 80 Strand, London WC2R 0RL, England

International Standard Book Number: 978-1-61564-795-8
Library of Congress Catalog Card Number: 2015930788

17 16 15   8 7 6 5 4 3 2 1

Interpretation of the printing code: The rightmost number of the first series of numbers is the year of the book's printing; the rightmost number of the second series of numbers is the number of the book's printing. For example, a printing code of 15-1 shows that the first printing occurred in 2015.

Printed in China

Note: This publication contains the opinions and ideas of its author. It is intended to provide helpful and informative material on the subject matter covered. It is sold with the understanding that the author and publisher are not engaged in rendering professional services in the book. If the reader requires personal assistance or advice, a competent professional should be consulted. The author and publisher specifically disclaim any responsibility for any liability, loss, or risk, personal or otherwise, which is incurred as a consequence, directly or indirectly, of the use and application of any of the contents of this book.

Most Alpha books are available at special quantity discounts for bulk purchases for sales promotions, premiums, fund-raising, or educational use. Special books, or book excerpts, can also be created to fit specific needs. For details, write: Special Markets, Alpha Books, 375 Hudson Street, New York, NY 10014.

PUBLISHER
Mike Sanders

ASSOCIATE PUBLISHER
Billy Fields

ACQUISITIONS EDITOR
Janette Lynn

DEVELOPMENT EDITOR
Kayla Dugger

DESIGNER
Rebecca Batchelor

PHOTOGRAPHER
Rebecca Batchelor

INDEXER
Johnna VanHoose Dinse

LAYOUT TECHNICIAN
Ayanna Lacey

PROOFREADER
Virginia Vasquez Vought

I would like to dedicate this book in loving memory of my grandmother Mary Klingler Hilliard, my grandmother Catherine Wilson, my sister Lori Klingler Chittendon, and my dear friend John Albinger. I feel all of you every day. Lastly, to my foundation, my concealer, my love ... Jay P. Langhurst.

CONTENTS

part 1
GETTING STARTED........3

1 TOOLS....................5
What You Need to Know
Before Buying Brushes 6
Five Must-Have Brushes................. 8
Other Brushes You Can Use 10
Disposables 13

2 SANITATION 15
Makeup Remover 16
Brush Cleaner 17
Maintaining Your Pencils and
Pencil Sharpener......................18
Getting Rid of Disposable Applicators....18
Disposal Dates.........................19

3 SKIN CARE.............. 21
Skin Types 22
Ten Power Foods for Healthy Skin....... 24
Cleansers............................ 25
Exfoliants............................ 26
Toners...............................27
Eye Creams 28
Moisturizers 29

part 2
BREAKING DOWN
YOUR LOOK 31

4 CORRECTIVE MAKEUP ...33
Analyzing Your Face 34
Using Highlight and Contour........... 38

5 FOUNDATION............43
How to Identify Your Skin Tone.......... 44
Types of Foundation.................. 46
Foundation Tools 50
Applying Foundation.................. 51

6 TINTED PRIMERS, CONCEALERS, AND TATTOO COVERS........53
Tinted Primer 54
Concealer............................ 56
Tattoo Cover 60

7 CHEEKS 63
Cheek Color Products................. 64
Highlighting and Contouring
Your Cheeks......................... 66
Applying Highlight, Contour, and
Blush by Face Shape................. 68

8 NOSE **73**

What You Should Know About
Your Nose 74

Nose Highlight and Contour
Shades and Tools 75

Highlighting and Contouring
Your Nose by Nose Shape 76

9 SETTING POWDER **81**

Types of Setting Powder 82

Powder Application Tools 83

Applying Setting Powder 84

10 EYEBROWS **87**

The Perfect Eyebrow 88

Eyebrow Types 89

The Best Eyebrow Types for Each
Face Shape 90

Brow Shaping 92

Filling in Brows 94

11 EYE SHADOW **99**

Types of Eye Shadows 100

Eye Shadow Finishes 101

Choosing an Eye Shadow Color 102

Applying Eye Shadow 101 104

12 EYELINER **107**

Types of Eyeliner 108

Basic Eyeliner Application 109

Going Beyond Basic: Eyeliner by Era 110

13 FULL EYE **113**

Parts of the Eye and Their Role
in Makeup 114

Correcting Your Eye Shape with
Full Eye Makeup 115

14 EYELASHES **121**

Types of Mascara 122

Mascara Colors 123

Mascara Wands 124

Basic Mascara Application 125

Other Eyelash Tools and Techniques 126

15 LIPS **133**

Lip Color Products 134

Choosing the Right Lip Color 137

Applying Lip Liner 138

Creating Balance Based on Your
Lip Shape 139

part 3
BRINGING YOUR LOOK
TOGETHER **143**

16 MAKEUP CHECKLIST **145**

Profile Sheet 146

Face Sheet .148

17 TEN CLASSIC LOOKS **151**

Daytime Natural 153

Elegant Evening 161

Dramatic Evening 171

1940s Bridal 181

1950s Chic 189

1970s Bronze 197

Metallic Smoky Eye 205

All About the Lips 215

Mature Mineral 223

Youthful Glitter 233

part 4
APPENDIX **241**

Glossary 242

Index 246

INTRODUCTION

Have you ever looked at a makeup application in a book or magazine or on the internet and attempted it, only to find it wasn't successful? Are you overwhelmed by all the makeup options at stores, to the point you don't know where to start? In *Idiot's Guides: Everyday Makeup Secrets*, I share all you need to know to create your best face, plus secrets on making your own products, fixing different makeup issues, and more. Whether your products and tools are high end or simply from your local drugstore, the tips and secrets I share with you will allow you to create a beautiful look you'll be happy to show off.

This book follows the principles of art and design, meaning each makeup application is defined by the art principles of color, shape, space, and form and the design principles of harmony, balance, proportion, and emphasis. So while there are many ways you can do your makeup, I focus on the tools and information you need to create the most flattering look on yourself.

To start, you get a primer on what you need before applying makeup—from getting and maintaining your makeup tools to prepping your skin. I've then broken down each feature by chapter so you can zero in on its role in your makeup and what you need to make it look its best. I close with 10 classic makeup looks you can try. From a natural look to a metallic smoky eye, these looks have stood the test of time and are varied enough that you'll be sure to find one you like. You can then use what you've learned about your unique features to translate any look to your own face.

Whether you read the book cover to cover or use it as a reference guide, I hope it helps to simplify makeup for you. Please feel free to reach out to me at neckupdesign.com if you have questions about a product or application. Most importantly, remember, it is not *makeup* that makes you beautiful; it is *you* that makes makeup beautiful!

ACKNOWLEDGMENTS

I have to start by thanking my childhood friend and acquisitions editor Janette Lynn. Thank you for trusting me with this book and for checking off the last box on my bucket list! Thank you to my editor, Kayla Dugger, for being so sweet and patient. Becky Batchelor (senior designer and photographer), thank you for working so hard and for being so excited about this project with me.

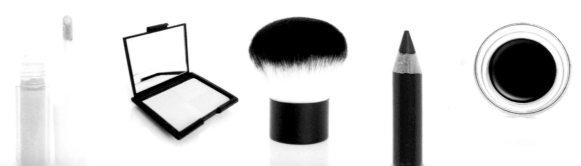

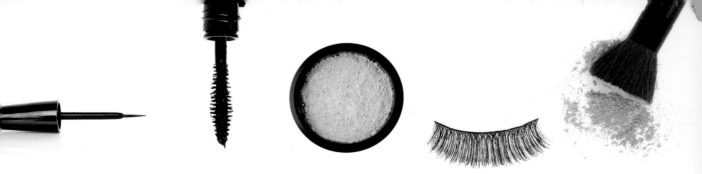

When creating a full-color book, one realizes they need back-up! This book went up another level with Lindsey Williams (crazypretty.com) as lead makeup artist. Lindsey, thank you for all of the phone conversations! Thanks to Ashley Heiney for saying yes when I asked her to assist with hair. And Carrie Duer, you're the best friend and personal assistant a guy could ask for! Thank you to my models: Josie Sanders; my beautiful niece Brooke Waltz; and my Indianapolis theater peeps, Betsy Norton, Cami Upchurch, Erin Coheneur, Arianne Villareal, Jill Kelly, Audrey Brinkley, Ashley Saunders, and Nathalie Cruz (who is currently in therapy for taking off her makeup so the readers could see what real people look like!).

I'd also like to give a special thank you to my clients and to the Indianapolis theater community. You have given me so much support and a space to learn and grow; I will forever be grateful. Thank you to my professional mentors Howard Leonard, Rosie Steffen, Susan Haise, David and Cathi Simon, Winn Claybaugh, and Debra Dietrich. Also, thanks to my parents Gerald and Sharon Kingler for giving me a great foundation.

Everyone needs a group of earth angels—people you can expose your heart to without judgment, people who will listen, people who will celebrate your achievements and hold your hand when you are in need, and people who truly exemplify unconditional love. I have always had that with Sarah Bernadette Ottow, Danya Sasada, Dana Nichols, Nora Crosthwaite, Laura Angel-Lalanne, Melissa Zabel, Margaret and Cameron Stutsman, and Phyllis Carr. Lastly, to Jay Langhurst, who says "no" so I have to prove him wrong! Love you most of all.

TRADEMARKS

PART 1
GETTING STARTED

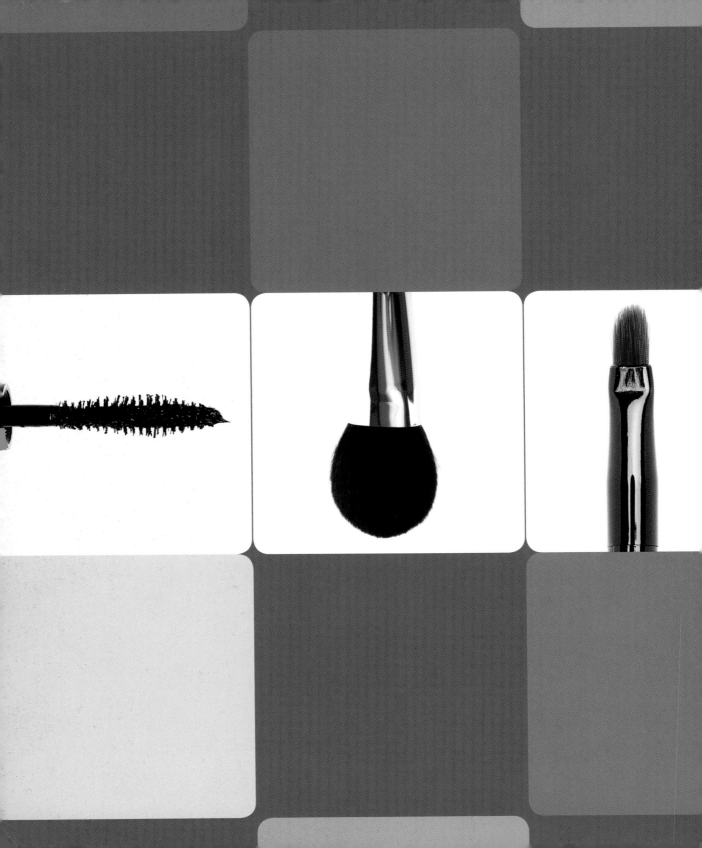

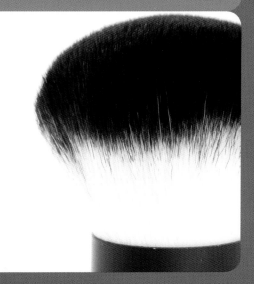

CHAPTER 1
TOOLS

The correct tools are a must in creating beautiful everyday makeup looks. For example, I can't tell you how many times I have watched my clients use the disposable applicator included with their eye shadow. That applicator should be thrown away the minute the eye shadow is opened! So it is my personal mission to get a set of brushes, as well as proper disposables, in every woman's arsenal.

In this chapter, I discuss makeup brushes, including what you must know before buying brushes, my five must-have brushes, and additional brushes you may want. I also take you through some handy disposable cosmetic tools.

WHAT YOU NEED TO KNOW BEFORE BUYING BRUSHES

Walking through a cosmetic store can be very intimidating.

There are a hundred different brushes that can be used for makeup application, many of which can be very expensive. However, you can find each of these tools at different price points depending on your budget. Just remember the adage "You get what you pay for"; investing a little more money in quality will provide savings in the long run.

Beyond price, there are four things you should consider when investing in brushes: fibers, density, ferrule, and handle.

FIBERS

Brushes are made from several types of fibers (bristles), which can be categorized as either synthetic or natural.

Synthetic fibers are animal fur free, which is what you'll get if you decide to purchase vegan brushes. Synthetic fibers are very soft, durable, and easily cleaned. This makes them ideal for applying cream makeup. However, they tend not to hold color pigments as well as natural fiber brushes.

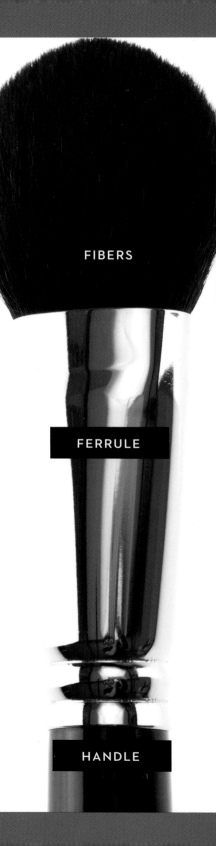

FIBERS

FERRULE

HANDLE

Natural fibers are made with animal fur. Goat hair is the most common in less-expensive natural fiber brushes and tends to be coarser. You can also find more-expensive brushes made from the fur of squirrels, badgers, horses, minks, and sable. Because natural bristles are more porous, they can be damaged by using cream makeup. Therefore, natural fiber brushes should only be used with powders.

DENSITY

Density refers to how many bristles are found in a brush head. Brushes that "dust" powder on the face, such as setting powder and blush brushes, do not require as many bristles. Brushes designed to deposit more color, such as kabuki and eye shadow brushes, should be denser.

FERRULE

The ferrule (pronounced like *feral*) is the metal portion of the brush that holds the bristles in place. Nickel is the most durable metal for your brush heads, so stick with that.

HANDLE

Makeup brushes are made with different handle lengths and material. Typically, a handle is either plastic or wood. Handles come in two lengths: short and long. Shorter handles are best when applying makeup on yourself, while longer handles are desirable when applying makeup on others. When it comes to material, a handle should be durable enough to withstand pressure and balanced properly for comfort and manipulation.

Brush Head Shapes

The shape of the brush head is another potential consideration when it comes to makeup application. The following are some examples of different types and what they're best for:

- **Round, fluffy, flat synthetic brush head:** This is great for blending and buffing foundation into the skin.
- **Soft, round, large natural brush head:** This can be used for dusting powder on your face.
- **Soft, medium-sized, dome-shaped natural brush head:** With this shape, you can apply blush and bronzer to the cheek area without disturbing the foundation.
- **Small, stiff, flat natural brush head:** This is ideal for applying eye shadows on the lid.
- **Flower-shaped, soft natural brush head:** The shape works to blend eye shadow on the lid. It is best used in circular motions.
- **Small-angled natural or synthetic brush head:** You can apply eyeliner and eyebrow colors with this type. Use the natural head with powders and the synthetic head with cream makeup.
- **Small, flat, round-tipped synthetic brush head:** This is best used to apply cream lip colors.

FIVE MUST-HAVE BRUSHES

There are many more brushes you can buy to make your application flawless. However, these five brushes are the basic tools I recommend to achieve your overall look.

1 POWDER BRUSH

A powder brush is the largest of the brushes you need. It is used to apply loose powder, typically after foundation is applied. A powder brush can also double as a tool to blend makeup.

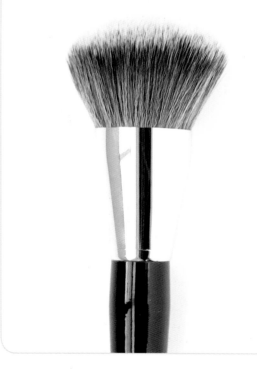

2 BLUSH BRUSH

A blush brush is a bit smaller than and not as full as a powder brush. Use the blush brush to apply cheek color powder (rouge or bronzer). You can also use this brush to apply contour color.

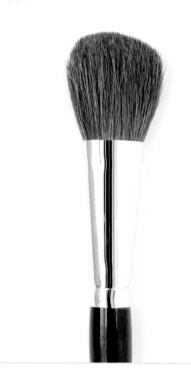

3 LARGE EYE SHADOW BRUSH

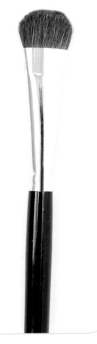

A large eye shadow brush made of either natural or synthetic bristles is great for applying lighter eye shadow pigments. I prefer a shadow brush with firm bristles, as I feel I have more control over the brush's placement and less drop-off (loose powder falling off the brush).

5 ANGLE BRUSH

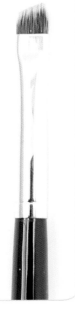

This brush is my favorite tool. An angle brush is flat, cut at an angle, and comes in both synthetic and natural bristles. You can use the angle brush primarily for eyebrow color and applying powder and gel liner around the eye.

4 MEDIUM EYE SHADOW BRUSH
(ALTERNATIVE: DOME EYE SHADOW BRUSH)

A medium eye shadow brush, made of either natural or synthetic bristles, is ideal for applying darker eye shadow pigments. Again, as a personal preference, I feel a firm bristle allows more control and distributes more shadow pigment; a brush with loose bristles does not hold as much powder.

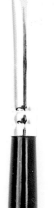

As an alternative to the flatter medium eye shadow brush, a dome shadow brush has dome- or round-shaped bristles and comes to a point. The dome brush fits into the crease of the eye. The point deposits stronger color into the crease, while the sides of the dome blend the color on either side.

Why Two Shadow Brushes?

I included two shadow brushes because, if you don't clean your brushes regularly, it keeps the application less muddy. The larger brush is good for applying the overall color of a lighter shadow, while the smaller brush is good for more detail and heavier, darker shadow.

OTHER BRUSHES YOU CAN USE

There are so many more brushes that assist in a flawless application.

It's important to understand what each brush does. The following are some brushes beyond my five must-haves you can use to apply your makeup.

LIP BRUSH

This brush is typically synthetic due to the fact lip colors are cream based. Its slanted edge can help you create a well-defined lip shape.

FOUNDATION BRUSH

A foundation brush is made from synthetic fibers and has a large head to help you cover more surface area on the face.

CONCEALER BRUSH

A concealer brush is made of synthetic fibers. Its small, thin size is perfect for applying concealer in smaller areas.

DUAL-FIBER BRUSH

A dual-fiber brush is made with a mixture of animal and synthetic fibers. It's a great brush to blend powder, liquid, or cream makeup, giving an air-brushed look to your makeup application.

BRONZER BRUSH

A bronzer brush is made from natural or synthetic fibers and has a dome-shaped head and dense bristles. As the name implies, it's used to apply powdered bronzer.

KABUKI (MINERAL POWDER) BRUSH

A kabuki (mineral powder) brush is typically short with wide, round or flat bristles. These bristles are dense to assist in applying a stronger amount of pigment.

ANGLED EYE SHADOW BRUSH

An angled eye shadow brush is perfect for applying color into the crease of the eye, due to its contoured shape.

FINE-POINT EYELINER BRUSH

A fine-point eyeliner brush is made from synthetic fibers and sometimes comes in an angled ferrule. Its thin, pointed head is great for detail work, making it useful for applying liquid and gel eyeliner.

SMUDGE BRUSH

A smudge brush can be made from either natural bristles or a sponge. This brush is designed to blend (smudge) a concentrated area, such as around the eye.

BLENDING BRUSH

A blending brush is made with natural or synthetic fibers, has a rounded head, and can sometimes be a little larger than a shadow brush. It's meant to blend shadow colors together, but you can also use it to add highlights to the cheekbones.

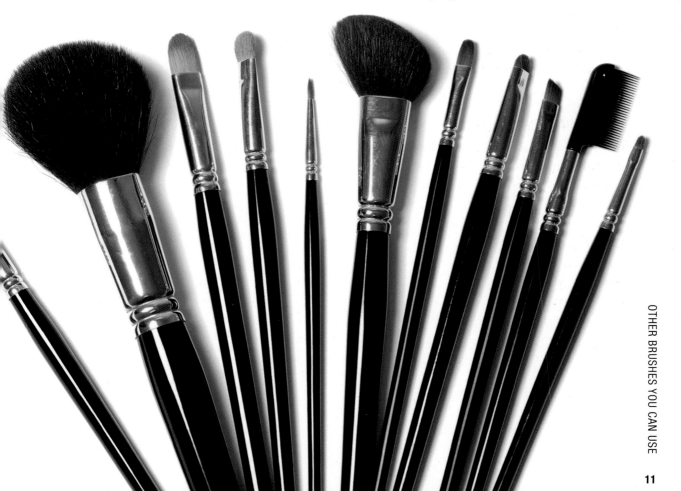

FAN BRUSH

A fan brush actually has several uses, including applying blush, blending powders, cleaning up excess powder, and highlighting the cheekbones.

BROW BRUSH WITH COMB

A brow brush with comb is made with synthetic bristles and has a plastic or metal comb on one end. This tool is designed to brush and comb eyebrow hair.

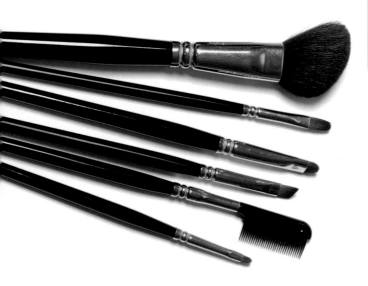

The Best Tools of All ... Your Fingers!

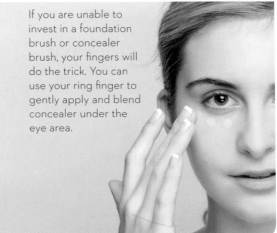

If you are unable to invest in a foundation brush or concealer brush, your fingers will do the trick. You can use your ring finger to gently apply and blend concealer under the eye area.

Beauty Sponges

Another handy tool for your arsenal is the beauty sponge, an applicator without edges that helps to distribute and blend makeup after application without the appearance of lines. Think of it as the difference between a paint brush (streaks) and a roller brush (no lines).

DISPOSABLES

To assist in your makeup application, I recommend using some disposable items along with your brushes.

These inexpensive disposable products can be found in any drugstore. They work in a pinch, are sanitary, and keep your applications neat and clean.

COTTON SWAB

Cotton swabs are great multipurpose tools when applying and correcting your makeup. You can use them to clean under the eyes where shadow or liner has smudged, clean around the lips, blend eye shadow, and apply lip gloss.

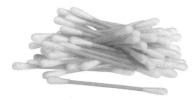

MASCARA WANDS

If you are in a family that shares makeup, you should invest in a box of disposable mascara wands. This will help you avoid any infections related to sharing the same wand for a product so close to your eyes.

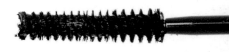

MAKEUP SPONGES

Makeup sponges, also called *wedges*, typically come in latex. Use these sponges to apply and blend foundation, to apply concealer, and to clean edges around the eyes and lips after makeup application. You can even cut makeup sponges in half to save on cost and waste.

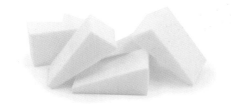

BABY WIPES

I always have a package of baby wipes on hand. They're great tools to use during application to clean the area where a mistake has occurred. In addition, baby wipes are a great alternative to the more costly facial wipes. They also have soothing agents, such as aloe, and are available in fragrance-free, hypoallergenic versions for sensitive skin. What's good for a baby's tender skin is ideal for your face!

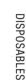

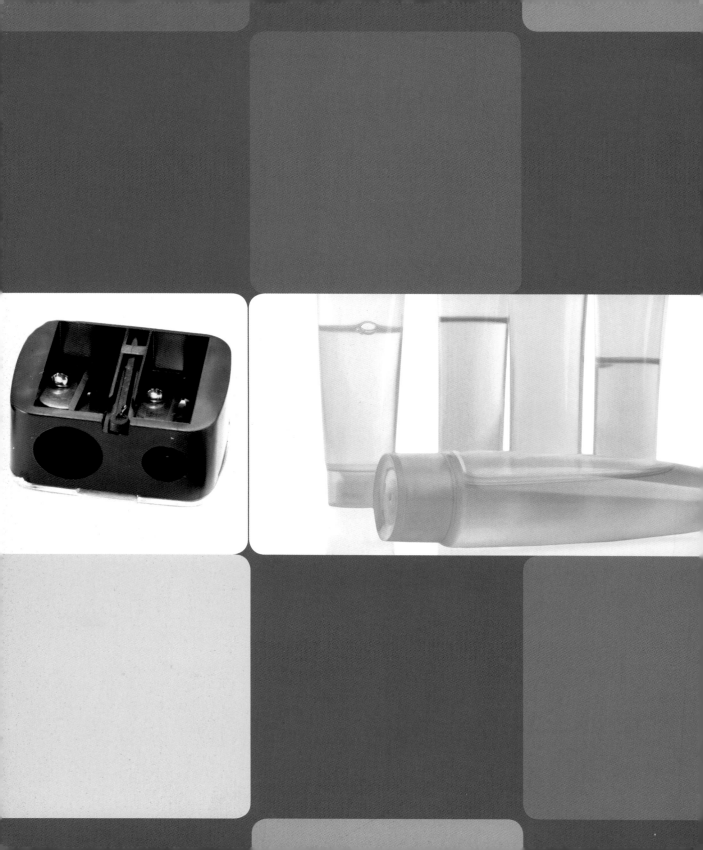

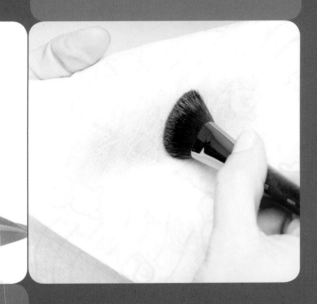

CHAPTER 2
SANITATION

Sanitation refers to the proper treatment of and disposal of tools. Over time, makeup products can become contaminated and harbor bacteria. Because your tools are moving from products to your face, it's important to take care of both your face and your tools. Therefore, it would be irresponsible not to discuss sanitation when it comes to makeup.

This chapter reviews cleanliness, how to take proper care of your makeup tools, and product expiration dates.

MAKEUP REMOVER

The last thing you want to do after a long workday or night out on the town is take off your makeup.

However, leaving your makeup on can clog pores, cause pimples and blackheads, and irritate the skin. It is very important to use a makeup remover prior to cleansing your face.

Makeup remover comes in three different types:

- **Makeup wipes:** Ideal for women who don't have the time (or patience!) for a lengthy cleansing regimen, these wipes are made of cloth dipped in facial cleanser. Once you've removed your makeup, you simply toss the whole wipe into the trash.

- **Oil-based cleansers:** Oil is an excellent ingredient to remove makeup, especially water-soluble products, because it dissolves the oil on your face without stripping away the natural oils your skin needs. Typically, oil-based products come in the form of creams and should be removed with cotton or a face towel.

- **Water-based cleansers:** These cleansers remove makeup and tone the skin, which returns the skin to its natural pH (4.5 to 5.5). They're a great choice for sensitive skin.

Water-based makeup removers work well for normal to oily skin, while oil-based cleansers work well for dry skin types. Whatever your skin needs, find a cleansing regimen that works for you, preferably with products that are fragrance, chemical, and alcohol free.

Creating Your Own Makeup Remover

Don't want to spend a lot of money on makeup remover? With a few inexpensive ingredients, you can create your own!

1 cup water

2 TB. baby shampoo

2 TB. extra-virgin olive oil

Combine water, baby shampoo, and extra-virgin olive oil in a jar or container and shake; this will help the oil and water come together. When you're ready to use the remover, apply it to a cotton ball and wipe it on your face.

BRUSH CLEANER

Makeup brushes pick up dead skin cells, dirt, oil, and product.

When you don't clean your brushes regularly, you are mixing debris into your products and onto your face. Therefore, you must clean your makeup brushes regularly to keep them sanitized.

The following are inexpensive tips to clean and maintain your brushes:

- In between uses, use a baby wipe to help remove leftover makeup on the brushes. I suggest using baby wipes that do not contain a lot of baby oil so you don't leave any oily residue on your brushes.

- Use dish soap and water to clean your synthetic brushes. Shake out any excess water and then lay them on a towel to dry.

- Because natural bristle brushes are similar to human hair, you can use shampoo and water to clean them. Once washed, shake out the excess water, form the bristles back to their original shape, and lay the brushes on a towel to dry overnight.

Creating Your Own Brush Cleaner

Because makeup brush cleaner can be expensive, here's a way to make your own.

½ cup dish soap

¼ cup extra-virgin olive oil

Pour dish soap and extra-virgin olive oil into a bowl. Swirl the brush in the mixture and rinse under warm water. Run the brush along your hand until the water runs clear. Shake out any excess water and lay the brush on a towel to dry overnight.

MAINTAINING YOUR PENCILS AND PENCIL SHARPENER

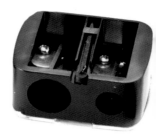

Your lips and eyes can contain debris and dead skin.

Therefore, always sharpen your cosmetic pencils after every use and be certain to return the lid to the product in order to keep your pencils clean.

Pencil sharpeners typically come with a dispenser to catch shavings. They are inexpensive and should be replaced once a year. However, you should still make sure to clean your pencil sharpener after you use it. To do this, empty the shavings and lead from the sharpener's inner compartment. Next, dip a cotton swab in isopropyl alcohol (rubbing alcohol) and work your way around the inside of the compartment, as well as the blade. The alcohol acts as a disinfectant. (You may want to use a toothbrush to remove cream from the pencils.)

Using the Correct Pencil Sharpener

Don't use a graphite pencil sharpener (used for number-2 pencils) on cosmetic pencils. They are not nearly as effective, plus any cross-contamination from regular pencils can lead to you getting wood shavings and graphite in your eyes. You can find sharpeners specific to cosmetic pencils in the beauty section of your local drugstore.

GETTING RID OF DISPOSABLE APPLICATORS

Cotton swabs, tissues, wooden spatulas, and cotton balls are examples of disposable applicators. All are great tools in helping you achieve your makeup look (or even removing makeup) without any special cleaning before or after. However, disposable applicators are not meant for multiple uses. They should be discarded upon completion of your makeup application.

2 SANITATION

DISPOSAL DATES

I am required, as a makeup artist, to invest in a vast assortment of makeup. So you can probably imagine the internal confict I go through when I decide to dispose of makeup.

Needless to say, all makeup comes with an expiration date. Your products contain preservatives that keep them from spoiling. Eventually, the products will begin to break down and can become contaminated.

Most cosmetic products contain a suggested disposal date. Therefore, if you aren't sure when to get rid of your product, look for the universal product expiration label on it. You should find a number indicating the length of time a product can be used (for example, 12m for 12 months).

Beyond that label, for safety and sanitation purposes, the following are the general recommended disposal dates for your makeup:

- **Mascara:** 2 to 3 months

- **Foundation:** 6 to 12 months

- **Eye shadow:** 12 to 18 months

- **Lipstick:** 12 to 18 months

- **Lip/eye pencil:** 18 to 24 months

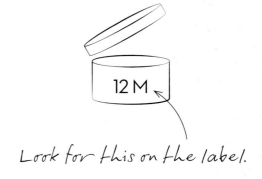

Look for this on the label.

Returning Makeup

Did you know that most drugstores and cosmetic counters will let you return gently used cosmetics? Save your money by returning makeup you can't or decide not to use.

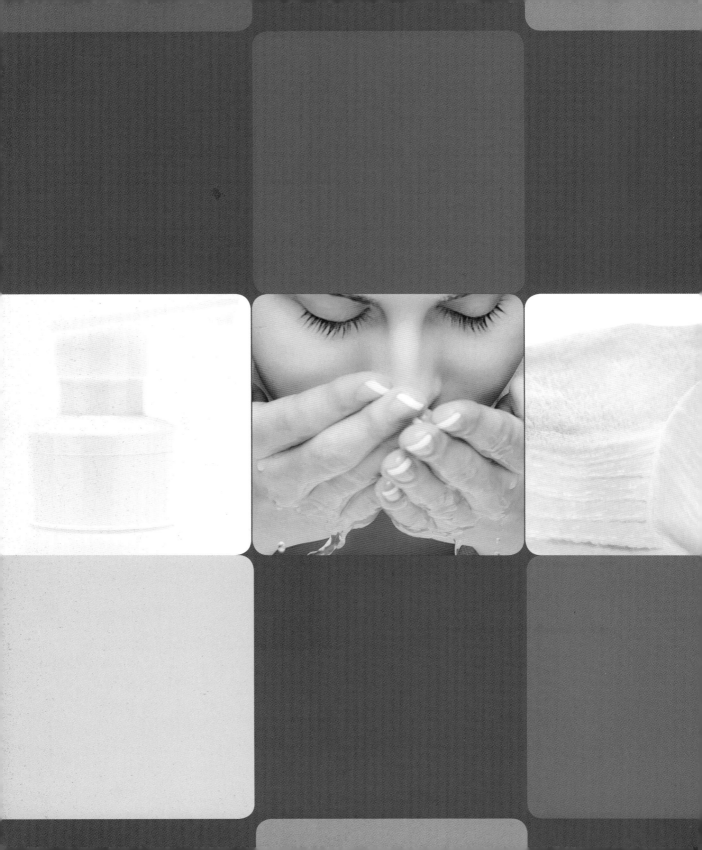

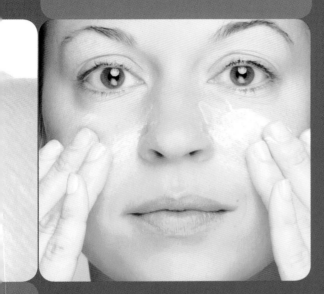

CHAPTER 3
SKIN CARE

Your face is the canvas to a beautiful makeup application. Therefore, in order to have people avoid painting on a dirty canvas, I always start my makeup consultations with a discussion about good skin care—and I'll do the same for you.

In this chapter, I help you first determine your skin type so you can know the products best suited for your skin. This chapter also discusses how what you eat affects your skin, as well as products you can purchase to support healthy skin.

SKIN TYPES

The first step to revealing your beauty through makeup application is good skin care.

To begin, you must determine your skin type to find the products best suited for you. Skin is generally classified into one of five categories: normal, oily, dry, combination, and sensitive.

NORMAL SKIN

Normal skin is the least problematic type of skin; it's not too dry and not too oily. Other characteristics of normal skin include the following:

- No or few imperfections
- No severe sensitivity
- Barely visible pores
- A radiant complexion

OILY SKIN

Oily skin can change depending on the time of year or weather. It is caused or made worse by stress, hormones, and/or exposure to heat or humidity. Other characteristics of oily skin are the following:

- Overactive sebaceous (sweat) glands
- Dull or shiny skin
- An excessive appearance of black-heads, pimples, and blemishes

DRY SKIN

Dry skin can crack; peel; or become itchy, irritated, or inflamed. If your skin is excessively dry, it can become rough and scaly, especially on the backs of your hands, arms, and legs. Other characteristics of dry skin include the following:

- Almost invisible pores
- A dull, rough complexion
- Red patches
- Less elasticity
- More visible lines

COMBINATION SKIN

Combination skin can be dry or normal in some areas and oily in others, such as the T-zone (nose, forehead, and chin). You will therefore need multiple products to address these different areas. Other characteristics of combination skin include the following:

- Overly dilated pores
- Blackheads
- Shiny skin

SENSITIVE SKIN

Skin can become sensitive for a variety of reasons. Most likely, it is caused by a cosmetic product, food, or your environment. You can attempt to eliminate products that cause sensitivity through trial and error. Otherwise, I encourage you to consult a dermatologist to diagnose the sensitivity. Other characteristics of sensitive skin include the following:

- Redness
- Itching
- Burning
- Dryness

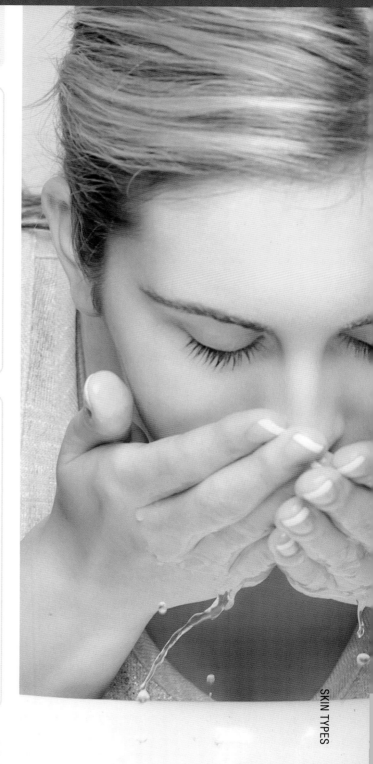

TEN POWER FOODS FOR HEALTHY SKIN

Diet is a large factor in the health of your skin.

As the saying goes, "you are what you eat." So before I get into skin care products, let's go over the 10 power foods that aid in skin health:

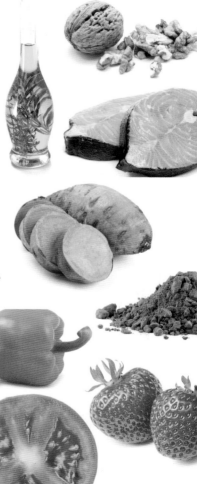

- **Cocoa powder:** This contains antioxidants that provide hydration. The caffeine in cocoa powder also benefits circulation in the skin.

- **Coffee:** You will find caffeine as an ingredient in many eye creams due to its anti-inflammatory effects. In the same way, drinking a cup of caffeinated coffee can help you reduce skin swelling and inflammation.

- **Fish:** Fish contain omega-3 fatty acids, which reduce inflammation. This makes fish a great diet staple for those with acne-prone skin.

- **Fruits:** Power fruits such as blueberries, oranges, and strawberries contain vitamin C, a super antioxidant. Vitamin C boosts the immune system, creates radiant skin, and helps blemishes heal properly.

- **Nuts:** Nuts contain protein, omega-3 and -6, vitamin E, calcium, and magnesium, all of which are good for fighting aging.

- **Olive oil:** Free radicals can lead to a loss of two things in your skin that keep you looking young: collagen and elastin. Olive oil has antioxidant polyphenols that help defend against these damaging free radicals.

- **Peppers:** The antioxidants in yellow and orange peppers help decrease skin's sensitivity to the sun, meaning fewer wrinkles!

- **Sweet potatoes:** These contain vitamin C, which smooths wrinkles by stimulating the production of collagen.

- **Tomatoes:** These are full of lycopene, a chemical that helps eliminate skin-aging free radicals caused by ultraviolet rays. Eating tomatoes also protects against sun damage.

- **Water:** Don't forget about H_2O! Six to eight glasses of water a day rejuvenate cell growth, making your skin look plumper and more hydrated.

CLEANSERS

Cleansers are essential in removing dirt and makeup so you have a fresh palette to work with.

It is recommended that you only wash your face twice daily—any more than that, and you strip your skin of its essential oils. Because there are many types of cleansers, I find it best to narrow down your choices by choosing a cleanser based on your skin type.

Normal: You can use most cleansers on this skin type. Specifically, cleansers that lather with water and cleansers without alcohol work best. Cleansers with alcohol can dry out your skin.

Oily: Cleansers that are water-based are great for oily skin. Look for cleansers that contain some type of acid, such as salicylic. This acid gently removes oil and reduces oil production.

Dry: Cleansers with moisturizers are ideal for dry skin types. Avoid using cleansers containing alcohol, as they can dry out your skin further.

Combination: The key to addressing combination skin is to identify cleansers that address the different problem areas. Foaming cleansers that are pH-balanced help correct combination skin. Avoid using harsh cleansers that may inflame areas of the skin.

Sensitive: Sensitive skin types have difficulty tolerating most cleansers due to the acids and strong detergents in them. Therefore, look for cleansers that are fragrance and preservative free. As in combination skin, you also want products that balance the skin's pH level.

Acne Cleansers

If you have acne-prone skin, look for cleansers that contain salicylic acid, which is a beta hydroxy acid used to treat acne. Cleansers specific to treating acne will be clearly marked that they help with acne-prone skin. Agents in these products assist in topical removal of bacteria and dirt and the cleaning of over-active sebaceous (sweat) glands.

EXFOLIANTS

Exfoliants are designed to remove dead cells from the surface of your skin. There are two types of exfoliants: mechanical and chemical.

Mechanical exfoliants contain abrasives such as microbeads, ground seeds, sugar, and salt. Almost any skin type can use a mechanical exfoliant. However, if you have sensitive skin, you may find this type of exfoliant to be abrasive.

Chemical exfoliants contain a lower concentration of "safe-to-use" acids. Chemical exfoliation is great for all skin types, but especially for those suffering with acne. This is because the acids used in chemical exfoliations go deeper into the skin, helping to unclog pores and reduce sebum (sweat) production.

Caution!

I strongly encourage you not to use exfoliants with microbeads on your face. One reason is they may create abrasions (cuts) in your skin. Another argument against microbeads is they are bad for the environment. If the product is not organic, the microbeads may be made from plastics, which can't be filtered during water treatment and will therefore cause them to wind up back in our lakes and oceans.

Lip Exfoliation

Did you know your lips also benefit from exfoliation? Removing debris and dead skin allows your lip product to adhere better and keeps lips healthy looking. One way to exfoliate your lips is with a soft or baby toothbrush. Another option is to use a lip scrub, which you can find in any skin care aisle. Whatever you decide, finish your exfoliation with a hydrating lip balm.

TONERS

I am going to be honest with you. For the longest time, I had no idea what a toner was or why I should use the product. Therefore, I'd like to share what I've learned with you so you know how important it is to use toner on your skin

Cleansers and exfoliants have an acid included as an ingredient. Acids (such as lactic or salicylic acid) are approved ingredients to gently remove dead skin, reduce oily skin, and unclog your pores. However, these acids change the pH of the skin, which is typically between 4.5 and 5.5, as you can see on the following scale.

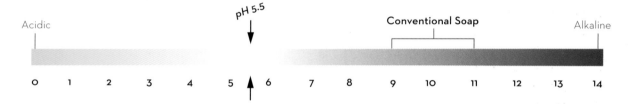

To leave the skin at a lower pH would cause the skin to dry. A toner is pH balanced to return skin to its proper pH level. Additionally, toners remove excess debris and reduce pore size.

Toner can be applied either by a spray mist or by using a cotton ball. I recommend applying toner after cleansing and exfoliation and before applying serums and moisturizers.

EYE CREAMS

Eye creams are used to reduce swelling, dark circles, and wrinkles.

The under-eye area contains much thinner skin and does not contain the sweat glands needed to keep the area moist. Therefore, it can be helpful to invest in an eye cream appropriate to your needs. As you mature, the collagen (which provides elasticity) begins to break down. Eye creams contain ingredients such as retinol to replace collagen and reduce the signs of aging.

The most common issues people use eye cream to combat are dark circles, puffiness, and fine lines and wrinkles. The following addresses the ingredients you should look for in an eye cream to treat those issues.

Dark circles: Contributors to dark circles include genetics, fatigue, broken capillaries, allergies, poor nutrition, age, and sun exposure. While a change of diet and lifestyle may still be the best way to combat or reduce dark circles in the long run, an eye cream that contains brightening agents like vitamin C, licorice, kojic acid, and niacinamide can help counter excess pigmentation and help stop the oxidation process that occurs on the surface of the skin. Retinols, peptides, and ceramides also work by thickening and strengthening the skin, making broken capillaries appear less visible.

Puffiness: While consuming salty foods and alcohol are the main reasons for puffiness under the eye, another way to combat this issue is to use an eye cream that contains caffeine. Most experts believe that caffeine stimulates circulation and constricts the blood vessels under the skin, diminishing the look of puffy eyes. As an antioxidant, it also protects the skin from sun damage.

Fine lines and wrinkles: If fine lines and wrinkles are your main concern, look for an eye cream that contains retinol, a powerful antioxidant embraced by dermatologists and estheticians alike for its ability to smooth lines and wrinkles. Aside from assisting in the production of healthy skin cells, retinol works by hampering the breakdown of collagen (a protein that gives the skin structure, firmness, and elasticity).

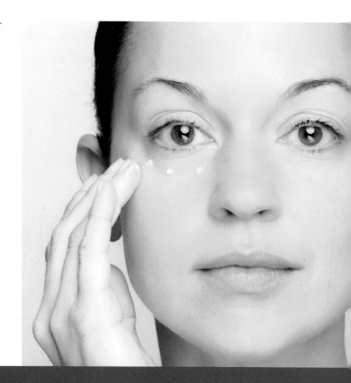

MOISTURIZERS

Once toning and exfoliation are complete, you finally can apply a moisturizer.

Moisturizers contain humectants (conditioning agents) that return moisture to the skin and help to keep water intact. Because removing makeup can be strenuous on the skin, finding the right moisturizer also helps to keep the skin healthy and fresh.

The table includes the composition of moisturizers you should look for based on your skin type.

Skin Type	Moisturizer
Dry skin	Heavier, oil-based moisturizers
Oily skin	Lighter, water-based moisturizers
Mature skin	Oil-based moisturizers
Sensitive skin	Moisturizers with soothing ingredients (such as aloe) that are fragrance and preservative free
Normal/ combination skin	Lighter, water-based moisturizers

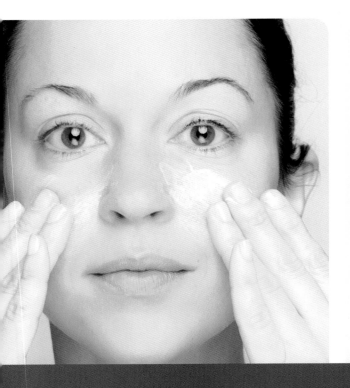

Moisturizers with SPF

Whenever possible, find a moisturizer with a sun protection factor (SPF). This refers to the theoretical amount of time you can stay in the sun without getting sunburned. For example, an SPF of 15 would allow you to stay in the sun 15 times longer than you could without protection. The SPF level needed depends on how fair your skin is—obviously the fairer you are, the higher the SPF you should go with.

By using a moisturizer with SPF, you're protecting against ultraviolet (UV) radiation, the skin's worst enemy. These invisible rays are part of the energy that comes from the sun and can damage the skin, potentially leading to melanoma and other types of skin cancer.

PART 2
BREAKING DOWN YOUR LOOK

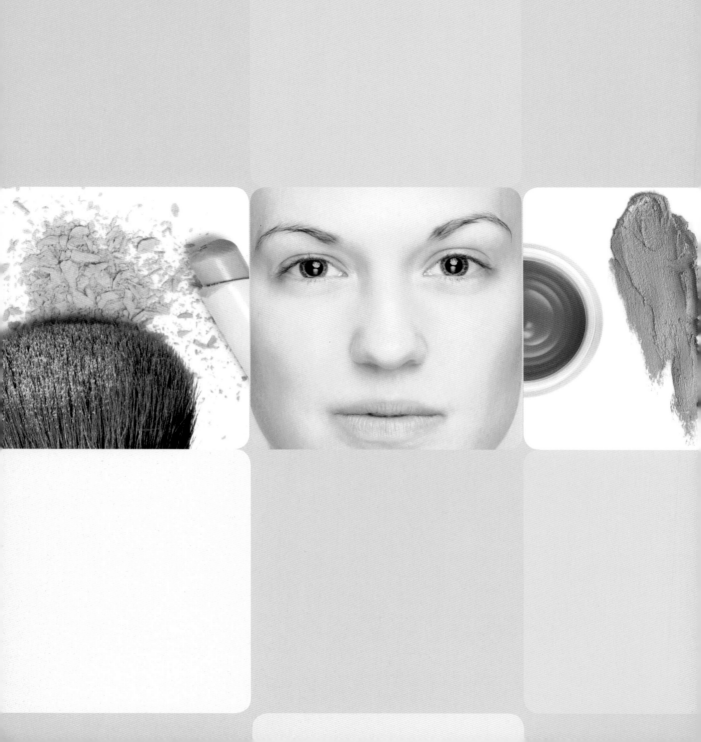

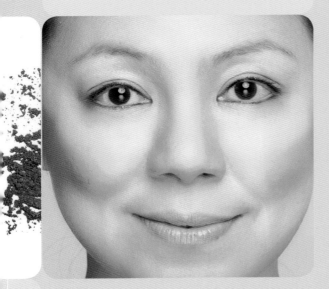

CHAPTER 4
CORRECTIVE MAKEUP

When decorating a house, an interior decorator must consider balance, scale, and proportion when planning furniture and accessory placement. These same principles apply to your makeup application. Corrective makeup is about moving your face toward the most attractive shape, balance, and proportion.

In this chapter, I first dissect the face and define its proportions. I then give you tips on how to highlight and contour your face to achieve the most desirable look.

ANALYZING YOUR FACE

Before you jump into applying corrective makeup to your face, it's important to know what "corrections" you need to make.

Beyond simple spot cover-up, corrective makeup is about achieving balance and proportion and giving your face an attractive shape. So let's take a moment to break down the face and its proportions.

THE THREE FACE SEGMENTS

The face is a three-dimensional object that can be divided into equal parts. The perfect face shape will have equal distance from the forehead to the eyebrow, the eyebrow to the tip of the nose, and the nose to the chin. The goal in corrective makeup is to create equality between these three segments using highlights and shadows for balance.

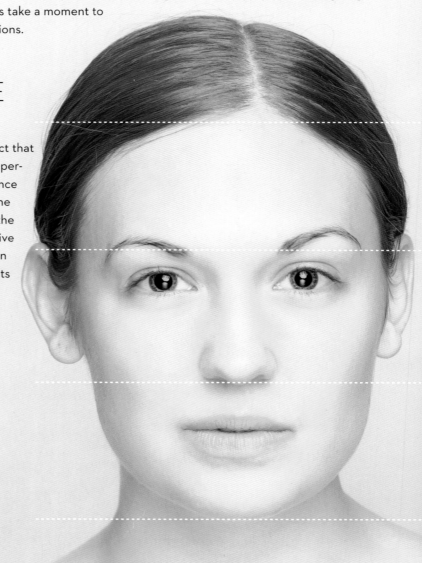

FACE PROFILE

Another part of the three-dimensional face is the profile. There are three face profiles: vertical, concave, and convex.

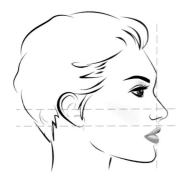 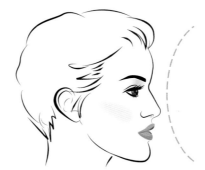 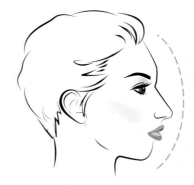

VERTICAL

This is the perfect face profile. The plane between the forehead and chin is straight up and down. This face profile does not require corrective makeup.

CONCAVE

This profile curves inward, making the forehead and chin more pronounced. You can create proportion within a concave profile by applying a contour color to the forehead and cheek. This will reduce and balance the profile.

CONVEX

This face profile curves out like a contact lens, while the forehead and chin slope inward and are less pronounced. By highlighting the forehead and the chin, you can create the illusion of harmony and proportion, creating a complementary relationship between the entire face profile.

WIDTH OF FACE

The perfect width of a face is three eye widths across. If you remove the third eye, you have the ideal spacing between the eyes. Corrective makeup will allow you to bring the eye shape inward using contour or outward using highlighting.

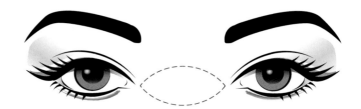

FACE SHAPE

The face shape is the surface of the front of the head from the top of the forehead to the base of the chin and from ear to ear. There are six different face shapes: oval, oblong, heart, diamond, square, and round. I'll discuss the characteristics of each face shape here; later, you'll learn how to highlight and contour by your face shape.

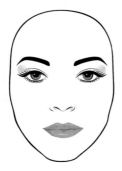

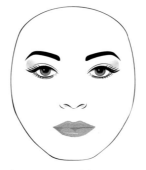

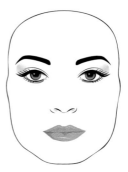

Oval: This is considered the most desirable and ideal face shape because it's a third less wide than it is long and doesn't have any major corners around the hairline or jawline. The oval face shape is round on top and curves down like an inverted egg.

Round: On a round face shape, the cheeks are the widest part of the face, with soft corners at the forehead and jawline.

Square: The width of the forehead, cheekbones, and jawline are equal on a square face shape.

The "Perfect" Face

During the European Renaissance, renowned artists and architects used an equation known as the "golden ratio" to map out their masterpieces. Thousands of years later, scientists adopted this mathematical formula to help explain why some people are considered beautiful. The golden ratio is a scale from 1 to 10 (with 10 considered the perfect face shape).

The first test is dividing the length of the face by the width. The ideal result—as defined by the golden ratio—is roughly 1.6, which means a beautiful person's face is about 1½ times longer than it is wide.

Next, the three segments of the face—from the forehead hairline to a spot between the eyes, from between the eyes to the bottom of the nose, and from the bottom of the nose to the bottom of the chin—are measured. If the numbers are equal, a person is considered more beautiful.

Finally, statisticians measure other facial features to determine symmetry and proportion. On a perfect face, for example, the length of an ear is equal to the length of the nose, and the width of an eye is equal to the distance between the eyes.

Worried you don't have what's considered the "perfect" face? There's good news. Scientists have never found a person with a perfect 10!

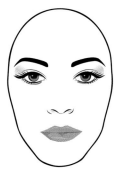

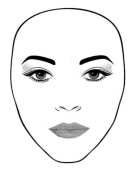

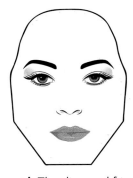

Oblong (Rectangle): This face is similar to a square; however, the oblong face shape is longer than it is wide.

Heart: Think about a heart and you'll understand what comprises this face shape. It is widest at the forehead and slightly less wide at the cheek, while the jawline is small and pointy.

Diamond: The diamond face shape has a narrow hairline and jawline and prominent cheekbones.

USING HIGHLIGHT AND CONTOUR

Corrective makeup is about simply using highlights (light) and contour (dark) to change the shape of the face.

Whether it's a crooked nose you would like to straighten, eyes you would like to emphasize, or a strong jawline you wish to soften, corrective makeup highlights features you find attractive and hides any features you find less flattering. While full corrective makeup is a bit more challenging and is not needed every day, knowledge of corrective makeup will be transformative.

The rule of thumb when doing corrective makeup on your face is to use a highlight one to two shades lighter and a contour one to two shades darker than your skin tone. If you'll be in a venue that's more dimly lit (such as a restaurant in the evening), you can go up to three shades lighter and darker respectively. (I will break down highlighting and contouring specific facial features in the following chapters.)

HIGHLIGHTING PRODUCTS

Highlighting is the process of lightening an area to bring it forward or make it more prominent. The following are products you can use to achieve a highlight on the face.

Powder: You can use a light matte powder or a light shimmering powder, whether pressed or loose, to highlight features.

Cream: You can find cream makeup in tubes, pencils, and pots. It is a great choice for highlighting, because it creates a dewy glow to the skin.

CONTOURING PRODUCTS

Contour is the use of shadows or shading to reduce features on the face. It's about the shade (slight degree of difference between colors) you use in contouring. In most instances, you will want to choose colors that are matte, as makeup with shimmer or glitter reflects light and draws focus to the area—the opposite effect contour is designed to achieve.

While many cosmetic companies have packaged "contouring" palettes, the following are some individual products you can use to contour.

Eye and cheek shadow: Matte shadows in shades of red, orange, and brown (depending on your skin tone) are popular for contouring. A pressed or loose shadow powder is a great choice for oily skin types.

Cream: Cream makeup is great for normal to dry skin types to use for contouring. Like eye shadow used for contouring, cream contour should be a shade of red, orange, or brown (depending on your skin tone).

Tinted powders: Tinted powders come in many contour shades. They are sheerer than a pressed powder, which can help you achieve a more natural look.

Bronzer: If you are trying to achieve a more sun-kissed look, you can use bronzer as a contour.

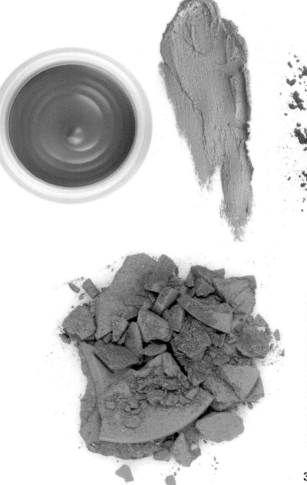

HIGHLIGHTING AND CONTOURING BY FACE SHAPE

Now that you know the parts of the face and what highlighting and contouring products you can use, it's time to learn how to highlight and contour based on your face shape. Remember, the goal of corrective makeup is to reduce or enhance portions of the face so they more resemble an oval, which is the ideal face shape.

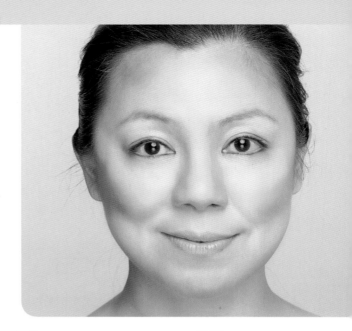

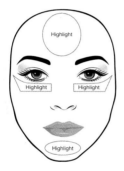

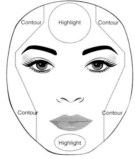

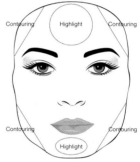

OVAL

Highlight: Apply highlight on the forehead, under the eyes, and on the chin. The highlights accentuate and brighten these areas of the oval face.

Contour: Contour is not needed since the oval is the ideal face shape.

ROUND

Highlight: Apply highlight to the center of the forehead and chin to bring the eye more to the center.

Contour: Apply contour to the jawline to reduce fullness and from the temple to the hairline to lessen the face's roundness.

SQUARE

Highlight: Apply highlight on the forehead and on the chin. This softens the strong lines of a square face.

Contour: Apply contour to both sides of the forehead and from the jawline to below the ear. This essentially reduces the "four corners" that create a square shape.

Identifying Your Face Shape

Still not sure what highlighting and contouring you need for your face? Here's quick and fun way to identify your face shape!

1. Stand in front of a mirror with overhead lighting, such as in your bathroom.

2. Pull your hair and bangs away from your face.

3. Using lipstick, quickly outline your face on the mirror (excluding the ears).

4. Step back and look at the shape.

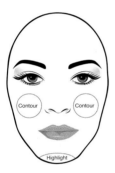

OBLONG (RECTANGLE)

Highlight: Apply highlight on the chin to attract attention to the center of the face.

Contour: Apply contour to the cheeks to reduce the length of the face.

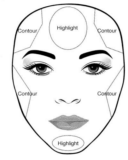

HEART

Highlight: Apply highlight to the center of forehead and on either side of the chin to give the face more fullness.

Contour: Apply contour at the corners of the forehead and to the cheeks to reduce their width. It should also be applied on the bottom of the chin to soften its pointiness.

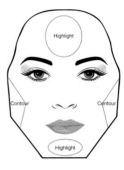

DIAMOND

Highlight: Apply highlight to the middle of the forehead and on the chin to emphasize the center of the face. Because the diamond face shape has pronounced cheekbones, however, it does not always need a highlighter.

Contour: Apply contour on the outside of the cheekbones to diminish their width.

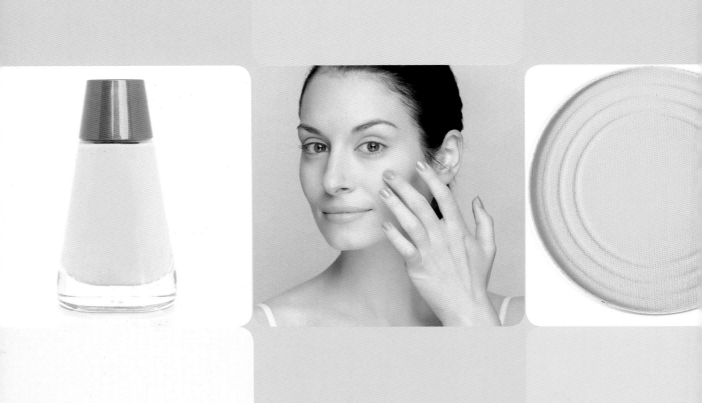

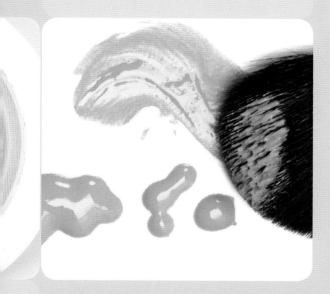

CHAPTER 5
FOUNDATION

Foundation is the first step to makeup application. It is skin-colored makeup used to even skin tone, cover skin flaws, and sometimes even change the color of the face. As its name denotes, it is laying the foundation for the entire application. That is why it's important to educate yourself on the correct product for you.

In this chapter, I discuss how to identify your skin tone, types of foundation and coverage, and how to apply foundation.

HOW TO IDENTIFY YOUR SKIN TONE

Human skin ranges from the darkest brown to the lightest pinkish-white.

Skin color is a result of the body's need to protect itself from UV rays. Skin color is affected by many substances, the primary one being melanin, which is a group of natural pigments found in most organisms. The level of skin pigmentation shows a close correspondence with latitude—people living near the equator tend to have dark skin, while light-skinned people mostly live nearer the poles.

Skin tone refers to the "undertone" or secondary color of the skin. It is not what you think of as fair, olive, tan, or dark; instead, it refers to the coloring under the skin. For example, someone who has fair skin might exhibit some redness in the skin; that redness is the undertone. You may have heard of your skin tone referred to in terms of being a Winter, Spring, Summer, or Fall tone. Currently, the terminology makeup artists use for skin tone is warm and cool; check out the following color chart to see what colors comprise these skin tones.

WARM
Yellow, peach, or golden tones

COOL
Pink, red, or blue tones

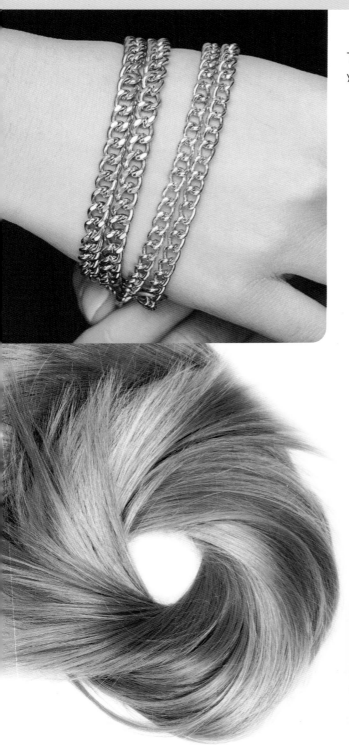

The following are some tests you can try to see if you are a warm or cool tone:

- Put on some jewelry or look at whatever jewelry you're already wearing. If you look better in gold jewelry, you most likely have warm undertones. If you look better in silver jewelry, you most likely have cool undertones.

- Look at the veins in your arms. If they appear greenish, you are likely to have warm undertones. If they appear blue, you have cool undertones.

- Your hair never lies! If you tend to pull more copper and gold tones in your hair, you are likely to have warm tones. If your hair is neutral to ash (blue) in color, you are likely to have cool tones.

- The clothes you look good in can also indicate your skin tone. If you look better in white or black fabrics, you are cool toned. If you look better in brown and off-white fabrics, you are warm toned.

- When you spend time in the sun, do you burn easily? If you do, you are most likely cool toned. However, if you tan easily, you are most likely warm toned.

Neutral Tone

Can't decide what your skin tone is based on these tests? You may just be neutral toned. People who have neutral tones look good in all colors, though they may personally favor the color palette of one tone over the other.

TYPES OF FOUNDATION

There are several types of foundation, and each works very differently on the skin to maximize its beauty.

The following table goes over the different attributes of each of the traditional types of foundation. Take a look and see which one you think would work best for you.

Type	Consistency	Coverage	Benefits	Finish	Skin Type	Application
Cream	Thick	Full	Covers birthmarks, pigmentation, acne, and scars	Matte	Normal, combination, dry, and mature skin	With a foundation brush, a sponge, or your fingers
Liquid	Thin	Medium	Covers flaws and provides hydration	Dewy and light	All skin types, especially dry and mature skin	With a foundation brush, a sponge, or your fingers
Pressed powder	Powder	Medium to full	Reduces shine and oil	Natural, even, and matte finishes	All skin types, especially oily	With a powder brush or sponge
Tinted	Half moisturizer and half foundation	Light to medium	Provides hydration and evens skin tone	Dewy and light	Dry and combination skin	With a foundation brush, a sponge, or your fingers

THE SPECIAL CASE OF MINERAL MAKEUP

Beyond the options I listed previously, you can also choose to use mineral makeup. Mineral makeup is comprised of all the same ingredients as regular foundation (mica, titanium oxide, zinc oxide, and iron oxides). However, it contains a light sunblock and anti-inflammatory properties and does not include parabens, preservatives, mineral oil, dyes, or fragrance, making it a healthy choice for the skin.

When concealing skin with minimal issues, I suggest you use a full-coverage foundation instead of a concealer; a full-coverage foundation will be less thick and more natural. Apply your foundation or concealer under your eyes and around the nose, and dab on blemishes or other small areas where you want full coverage. You can then apply your mineral foundation makeup (with a foundation brush or kabuki brush) all over your face. Blend the mineral makeup into the areas that you want concealed, and finish your look by spraying your face with a hydration mist. Your result will be beautiful, natural-looking skin.

If you would like to learn how to make your own mineral makeup, check out *Idiot's Guides: Making Natural Beauty Products*.

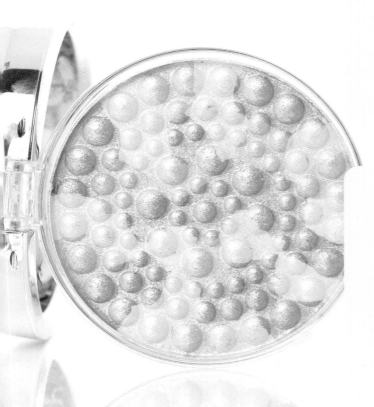

Did You Know?

While mineral makeup originally started out as a loose powder, you can now buy mineral makeup in beautiful eye shadows, blushes, and bronzers.

Using a Kabuki Brush for Mineral Makeup

A kabuki brush is a brush specifically made for the application of mineral makeup. With its short handle and dense bristles, it is designed to hold more powder for more coverage.

LEVEL OF COVERAGE

Another thing you should consider when choosing foundation is the level of coverage you'd like. There are three types of foundation coverage: sheer to light, medium, and full.

Sheer to light coverage: This type of foundation coverage is lightweight and transparent, with very little coverage. It evens skin tone; however, this won't cover flaws.

Medium coverage: With this type of coverage, you can reduce the appearance of small blemishes and uneven skin tone. However, it won't completely disguise the skin from its natural color and imperfections.

Full coverage: This type of coverage completely covers flaws and uneven skin tone. However, it can clog pores and may encourage skin breakouts.

Choosing the Right Foundation

When choosing a foundation, test the foundation on your neck leading into your jawline rather on your face. Your face can easily be a different shade than the rest of your body due to sun or irritation, so the goal is to match your face with your body. A good rule of thumb is to go slightly darker rather than lighter in color if you have a fair to medium skin tone in order to avoid looking like you have a "mask" on. On the other hand, if you have a darker skin tone, use a foundation slightly lighter than your natural skin tone to brighten your face and allow your makeup application to stand out.

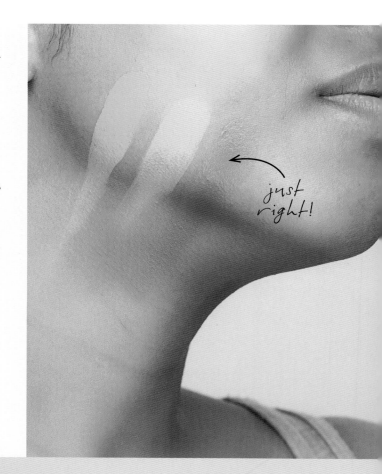

just right!

FINISHES

Foundations come in three types of finishes, which can alter the look of your skin: matte, shimmer, and dewy.

Matte: Foundation with a matte finish does not contain a reflecting agent. This makes it the best product to use when contouring your face.

Shimmer: A shimmer finish foundation contains reflecting agents that draw attention to your makeup, creating a more dramatic look. Because shimmer foundation reflects light, it can be used as a highlighter above the cheekbone to the temple.

Dewy: Foundation with a dewy finish contains moisturizers to create a fresh, youthful, and luminous look. If you have mature or dry skin, it can also be used to make your skin look more hydrated.

Making Your Own Tinted Moisturizer

To create your own tinted moisturizer, place a little concealer with a quarter-size amount of your favorite facial moisturizer on your hand. Mix with your fingers or a cotton swab and then apply to your face. Voilà, tinted moisturizer!

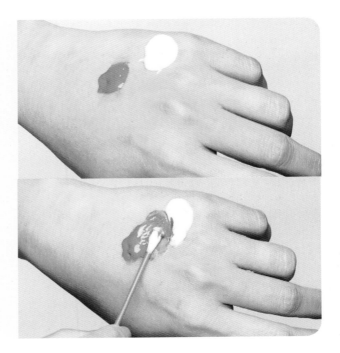

FOUNDATION TOOLS

There are three primary tools you can use to apply foundation: a sponge, a brush, or your fingers.

Whatever you decide to use, apply the foundation in downward strokes to avoid elevating your fine facial hair.

SPONGES

The most common types of makeup sponges are latex and natural sponges. Latex sponges are disposable and are only good for one-time application, while natural sponges (such as sea foam) are designed for multiple-use applications. Both types of sponges can be used for both dry and damp foundation application. Additional benefits of using a sponge include more control of the product, a sheer and lightweight application, and an inexpensive investment.

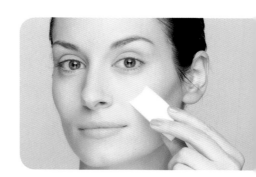

BRUSHES

I like to think of a foundation brush as a "paint brush." A foundation brush has a larger head, allowing for more coverage during application. Its bristles are also synthetic, which allows for easy cleaning. The benefit of applying foundation with a brush is that it keeps the spread of bacteria (and therefore acne) to a minimum. While this brush may cause some streaking, you can stipple or tap your brush over the foundation to have a more even application.

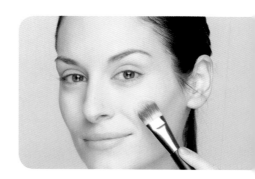

FINGERS

Fingers are the best tools you have at your disposal! Using your hands and fingers allows you to feel and control the application of foundation, leading to better blending.

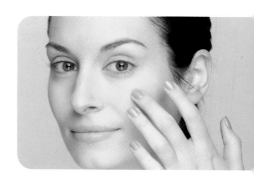

APPLYING FOUNDATION

The following walks you through how to best apply foundation.

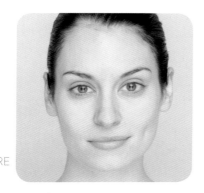 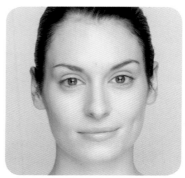

BEFORE   AFTER

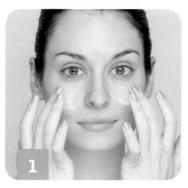 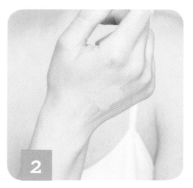 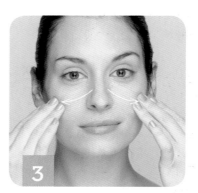

1. Before you apply your foundation, moisturize your face. If you recall from my discussion of skin care, foundation will go on much more evenly when the face is moisturized.

2. Apply foundation to the back of your hand. Your hand will warm up the foundation, allowing it to go on more smoothly.

3. Swiping the foundation off your hand, start applying in the center of your face (the sides of your nose) and work outward. Blend the foundation evenly throughout your face, paying close attention to discolored areas of the face that may need a bit more foundation.

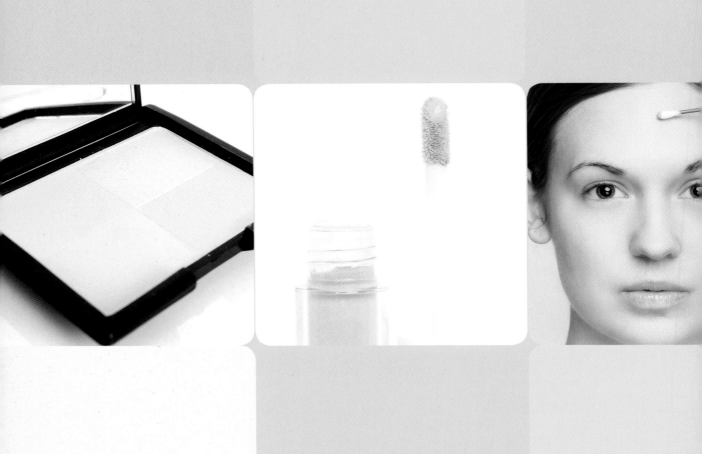

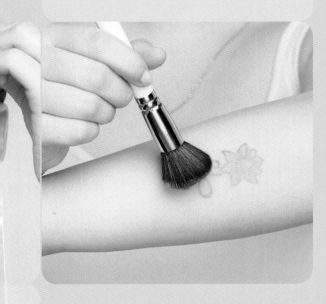

CHAPTER 6

TINTED PRIMERS, CONCEALERS, AND TATTOO COVERS

Primers, concealers, and tattoo covers are designed to provide the coverage foundation cannot. While foundations assist in changing overall skin color and evening out skin tone, in some instances, blemishes, dark circles, and even tattoos can't get the coverage they need. Tinted primers are applied first to improve coverage of your makeup and its duration. Concealers can then be used to cover dark circles, discoloration, age spots, and blemishes. And if you need to cover up a tattoo, tattoo covers give you the thickness and coverage you need.

In this chapter, I discuss the products and application in regard to tinted primers, concealers, and tattoo covers.

TINTED PRIMER

A cosmetic primer is a cream or lotion applied before concealer and foundation; think of it as priming a wall for painting.

Through this, you can help reduce creases in your makeup and the visible signs of crow's feet. Primer also removes color so the shades you want to achieve will be more successful. There are primers for the eyelids, face, and lips that are used to address discoloration from under-eye circles, blemishes, scars, and so on.

If you are experiencing discoloration and dull or lifeless skin, tinted primers may be a great choice for you. These come in shades that follow the law of complementary colors (other than neutral). For example, if the color is red, its complementary color is green. If you mix red and green together, you get a shade of beige/brown. Consequently, if your blemish is red and you apply a green primer, you will neutralize the color to beige.

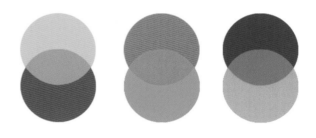

How Much?

Just a dab will do you! You need only to apply the smallest amount of primer to achieve the proper results. If you apply too much, you may struggle with neutralizing the pigment.

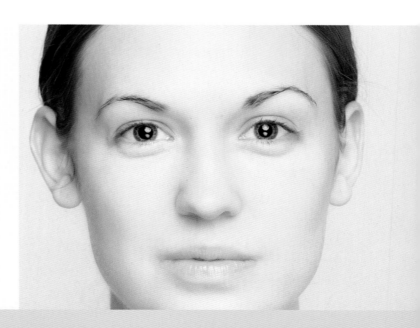

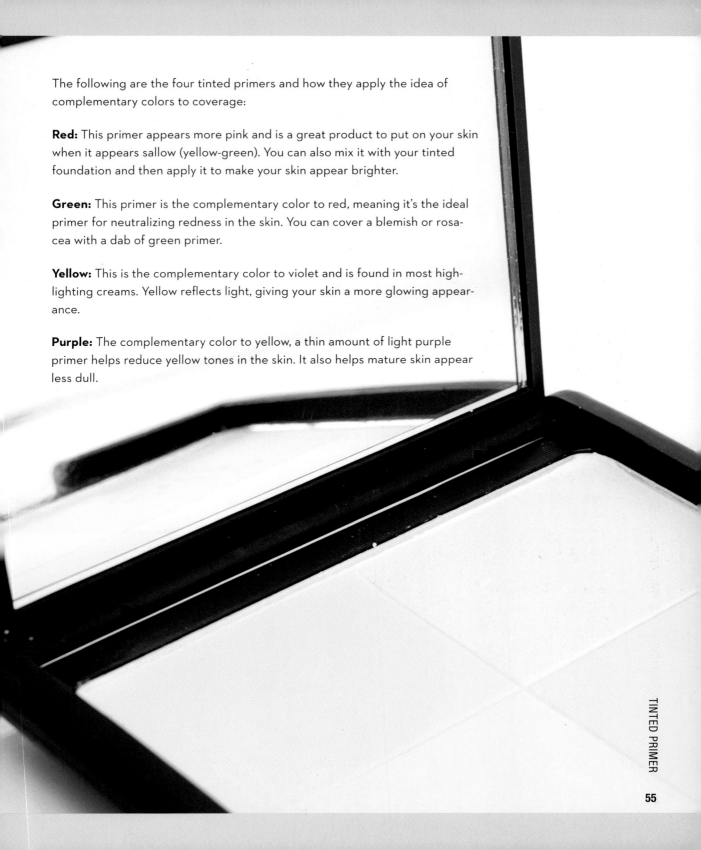

The following are the four tinted primers and how they apply the idea of complementary colors to coverage:

Red: This primer appears more pink and is a great product to put on your skin when it appears sallow (yellow-green). You can also mix it with your tinted foundation and then apply it to make your skin appear brighter.

Green: This primer is the complementary color to red, meaning it's the ideal primer for neutralizing redness in the skin. You can cover a blemish or rosacea with a dab of green primer.

Yellow: This is the complementary color to violet and is found in most highlighting creams. Yellow reflects light, giving your skin a more glowing appearance.

Purple: The complementary color to yellow, a thin amount of light purple primer helps reduce yellow tones in the skin. It also helps mature skin appear less dull.

CONCEALER

Concealer is a flesh-toned cosmetic product that's similar to foundation but thicker.

I consider it to be one of the most important steps in makeup application. It would be a mistake to think of concealer simply as a "cover-up." Instead, think of concealer as a play on light and a manipulation of color. For example, if you are trying to cover dark circles (a shade or two darker than your skin color), you need to find a concealer that is a shade or two lighter than your actual skin color to counterbalance the discoloration.

TYPES OF CONCEALER

Concealer is full-coverage makeup that comes in liquid, cream, and powder form. Each can benefit your skin in different ways.

Liquid: This is great for dry skin, has a lighter finish, and is great for hydration. Liquid concealer can be used anywhere you need to cover imperfections. Additionally, it hydrates the under-eye area while reducing the look of dark circles and discoloration.

Cream: Much thicker than liquid concealer, you use a cream concealer when you have dark circles, pimples, scars, and bruises.

Powder: Typically found in the mineral makeup line, this type of concealer is great on oily skin. Powder concealer is best used when you are experiencing a little discoloration or a small skin imperfection.

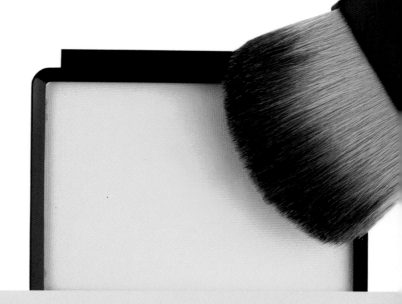

CONCEALER PACKAGING

You can find concealer in the form of sticks, compacts/containers, tubes, or pencils. The packaging is designed to assist you in easy application and spot treatment. The following is what typically comprises each type of concealer package.

Stick: Cream concealers typically come in a thin stick. They have a cream consistency and are good for covering blemishes.

Compact/container: Cream and powder concealers may come in a container, either as a compact or a container with a lid.

Tube: Liquid concealers come in a tube. You can either squeeze the product out or use an applicator that is included on the tube (like you would see on a lip gloss tube).

Pencil: Pencil concealers are thicker products that come in a pencil form. They are great for spot treating areas and for concealing your lips. Be careful when applying it under the eyes, however, since the skin there is thinner and requires a lighter touch.

Color-Correcting Concealer

Color-correcting concealer is a last resort when flesh-tone concealer doesn't work well enough to cover or neutralize severe discolorations. It is most commonly available in cream or stick form and is a thicker consistency than a tinted primer (which tends to be liquid and go on more sheer).

If you decide to try a color-correcting concealer, apply it before your foundation; this helps to neutralize and balance the unnatural color of it. You also can pair it with a flesh-tone concealer with the same finish, so that when the foundation is applied on top, there is no indication of the color corrector underneath.

The following are the different color-correcting concealers and what they correct depending on your concern:

- **Lavender:** Counteracts sallow or yellowness in the skin
- **Yellow:** Counteracts deep purple tones, such as dark circles or scarring; also works well to highlight brows and cheekbones when pale yellow
- **Green:** Neutralizes redness, including diffuse redness from rosacea
- **Pink:** Neutralizes a blue cast on lighter skin tones; can enliven very pale skin
- **Orange/salmon:** Neutralizes blue to deep purple or grayish tones on deeper skin tones

APPLYING CONCEALER

Typically you apply concealer under the eyes and around the nose and mouth. Additionally, you can use concealer to conceal blemishes, scars, and bruises. The following are some helpful tips on the best ways to apply concealer.

- Apply concealer under the eye with your ring finger, which tends to have the lightest touch. You can place it right below the tear ducts by tapping it lightly in a U-shaped pattern from the inside to the outside of the eye.

- Use an angle or eyeliner brush to dab concealer onto the top of any blemishes. Doing so helps to concentrate the product on top of the blemish.

- To reduce the look of puffy eyes, use a hydrating (liquid) concealer two shades lighter than your skin tone and apply it under the eye with your ring finger, a brush, or a beauty sponge.

Other Concealer Tips and Tricks

Concealer can be your best friend. Here are some concealer secrets to assist in making your application flawless!

- **Are you having a difficult time covering your dark under-eye circles?** Use a hydrating eye cream to plump up the under-eye area before applying your concealer.

- **Want to get rid of those fine lines?** All you need is a wrinkle-filling serum and some liquid concealer. Squeeze a bit of the wrinkle filler onto your finger, dab it into the wrinkle, and blend until it is barely noticeable. You can then top with the liquid concealer to completely hide that fine line.

- **Experiencing problems with covering uneven skin tone?** You don't want to overdo the concealing when you have uneven skin tones; otherwise, it can look extremely unflattering and unnatural. So start with your full-coverage foundation and place it on with a clean foundation brush or sponge. From there, dot on your yellow-based concealer and blend!

- **Would you like to wear that fabulous skirt, but you're afraid to expose those pesky spider veins on your body?** Use a pencil or wand-style concealer (in your skin tone) that will allow for the most coverage and control and trace over the veins. Blend the concealer with your pinkie finger and set with some pressed translucent powder!

- **Do you have a red and irritated nose due to a cold or allergies?** To get rid of the redness first, avoid a moisturizer; instead, just use a flat-tipped concealer brush or Q-tip with a bit of yellow-based concealer right around the red areas of your nose. Next, really blend on your foundation to neutralize the rest of the redness. Finally, cover it up with a bit of translucent powder!

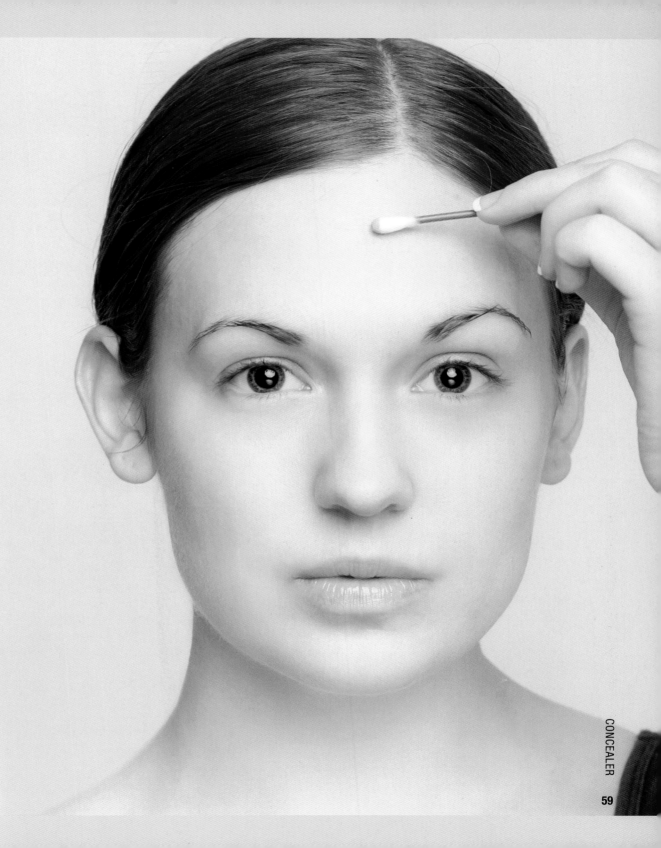

TATTOO COVER

Have you ever tried to cover a tattoo for a wedding or a formal function?

Foundations and concealers don't work well because they are usually sheer, slightly translucent, and simply won't cover the ink.

When you need to cover a tattoo, the product you want to use is tattoo cover (sometimes called *camouflage* cover). Tattoo cover has the same effect as a concealer, with the main difference being simply thickness. Tattoo cover is very thick with a matte finish to cover up the dark and multicolored inks used in tattoos. Stores sell tattoo wheels or palettes with multiple shades. Because skin isn't typically one color, the multiple shades are helpful in creating a more realistic look for your skin.

Ready to try covering your tattoo? The following walks you through how to do so.

Can't Find Tattoo Cover?

If you do not have access to tattoo cover, you can use a full-coverage foundation or even theatrical makeup. However, you may need a few extra coats to achieve the same coverage.

What You Need

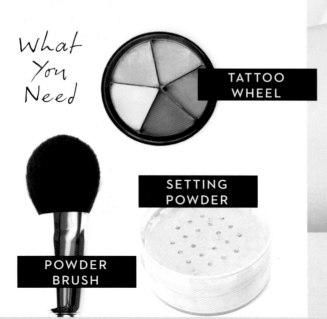

TATTOO WHEEL

SETTING POWDER

POWDER BRUSH

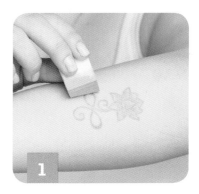

1

Choose a shade lighter than your skin color and press the cover-up into the area. You do not want to rub or brush the product into your skin, as it will move the product around, making it difficult to fully cover the tattoo.

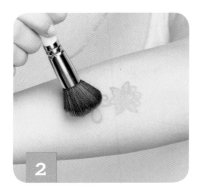

2

Use a setting powder to set the tattoo cover. If you can still see the tattoo, repeat covering the tattoo with the same shade of tattoo cover and then set with powder.

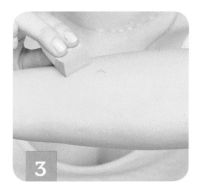

3

Choose three different-color shades of tattoo cover—one closest to your skin color, one slightly lighter, and one slightly darker. Using your fingers or a porous sponge, tap the shades over the area of your tattoo. This will replicate the different tones in the skin. Powder the area and repeat the process of tapping in the color shades as many times as necessary. Once you are left with a circle of product on your tattoo, blend the edges of the tattoo cover into your skin to even it out.

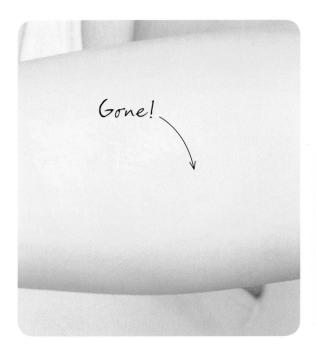

Gone!

Liquid Skin

Liquid Skin is typically used as a liquid bandage, but it also works well in enabling tattoo cover application. You can apply a thin layer of it over your tattoo and allow it to dry before following the steps for covering your tattoo. Liquid Skin is available in the first-aid section of your local drugstore.

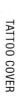

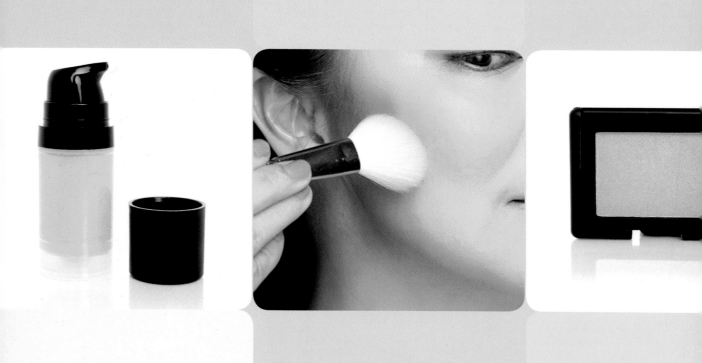

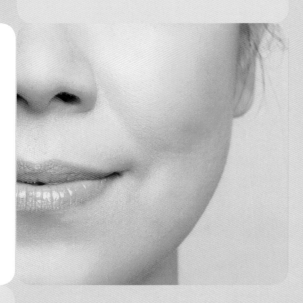

CHAPTER 7
CHEEKS

The cheeks are an important aspect of a makeup look. Cheek color can add a glow, change the face shape, and create drama. Everyone has the right to have amazing cheekbones! Do you feel you have nonexistent cheekbones? Are you uncertain about which cheek color is right for you?

In this chapter, I discuss the different cheek color products available, as well as how to create beautiful cheekbones based on your face shape and through the application of highlight, contour, and cheek color.

CHEEK COLOR PRODUCTS

Cheek color comes in several different shades, typically ranging in the red and orange families.

This pop of color can provide a healthy glow and give your face more balance. You can find cheek color in cream, powder, or mineral forms. Take a look at each type and see which is right for you.

Choosing the Right Color for Your Cheeks

Cheek color comes in warm and cool, so when picking out a color, consider your "undertone," as discussed in Chapter 5. The wrong color could make or break your final look. A good rule of thumb is to match your cheek color to your lip color.

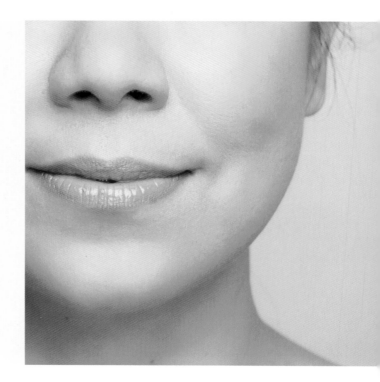

Cream: This type of cheek color goes on sheer and provides a dewy look to the cheek. It should be applied with a synthetic blush brush, a sponge, or your fingers. You should use cream color if you have normal or dry skin.

Powder: This cheek color tends to be more matte in finish and is applied to the cheeks with a blush brush. Powder cheek color is great for oily skin.

Mineral: This cheek color, applied with a blush or kabuki brush, is easy to blend with mineral foundation. It goes on sheer and illuminates the cheeks. Mineral cheek color is good for all skin types, especially sensitive and mature skin.

Bronzer: This type of cheek color provides a natural, sun-kissed glow without exposing your skin to the sun's harmful UV rays. Bronzer comes in cream, powder, and mineral forms (depending on your skin type). Matte bronzers also make an excellent contour. Depending on its consistency, you can apply bronzer with a blush brush, a sponge, or your fingers.

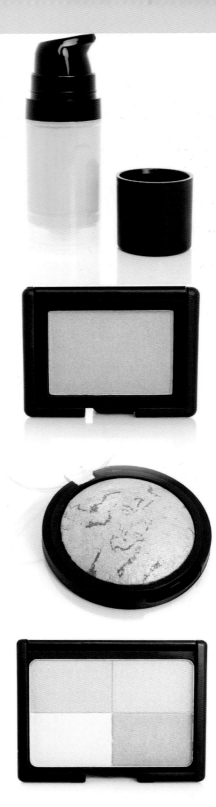

HIGHLIGHTING AND CONTOURING YOUR CHEEKS

If you choose to contour anything on your face, I would consider the cheeks to be at the top of the list.

A great cheek/cheekbone changes your face shape and directs the emphasis to the middle of your face. Plus, if you think your face is too round or your cheeks are too plump, you can rectify any problems and get the "supermodel cheeks" you crave. To change the shape of a cheekbone, similar to what you've learned with corrective makeup, you need a lighter shade (highlight) and a darker shade (contour).

Highlight: Because highlighting creates emphasis to the area, your highlight color should be a half to full shade lighter than your skin tone. Highlight colors come in powder and cream.

- *Powder highlight* is a great choice for those with oily skin. Some products may include a shimmer for additional glow.

- *Cream highlight* provides more hydration for those with normal to dry skin. Cream highlights naturally look shinier than powder, which makes them a great choice for a highlight.

Contour: Because contouring creates a shadow effect, your contour color should be a half to full shade darker than your natural skin tone. You can use either matte powder or matte cream.

- *Powder contour* is a great choice for those with oily skin and goes on matte.

- *Cream contour* provides more hydration for those with normal to dry skin. Cream contour is also easy to blend.

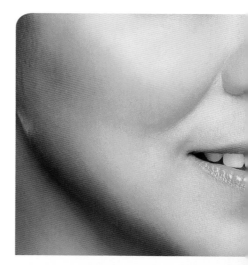

Cheeks in High Definition

Mix a cream cheek color with a little of your foundation and then apply it to your cheeks. The cream color will blend better with the foundation, giving your face a more uniform look.

If you choose to change the shape of your cheeks, you can follow these three easy steps.

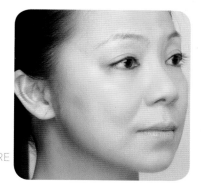
BEFORE

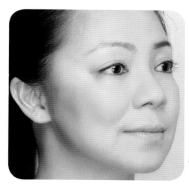
AFTER

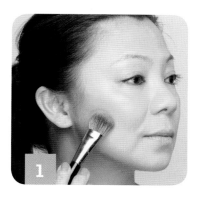

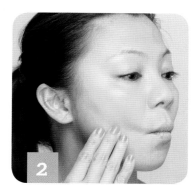

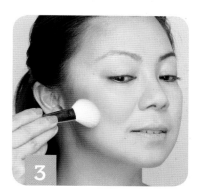

1. Look into the mirror while you suck in your cheeks. With a blush brush, apply your contour between the bottom of the cheekbone and above the jawline. This helps to reduce the area of the cheek you want to appear slimmer.

2. Take your fingers and feel your cheekbone start under the center of your eye and moving back to your temple. Add a light powder or cream as a highlight to make this area more prominent. This also brightens the eye area while providing definition.

3. Apply your cheek color between the highlight and the contour, and then blend all three together.

APPLYING HIGHLIGHT, CONTOUR, AND BLUSH BY FACE SHAPE

Now that you know about how to highlight and contour your cheeks, as well as change the shape of your cheeks, it's time to bring these together.

The following shows you how to apply highlight, contour, and blush based on your face shape.

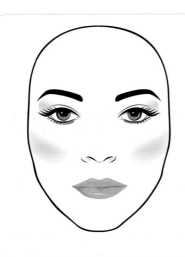

OVAL

Remember, oval is the ideal face shape. Therefore, highlight and contour will not be needed unless you want to accentuate the hollows of the cheeks or upper cheekbones. The ideal placement of cheek color would be to apply the blush across the cheekbones; however, keep it to just under the outside of the eye, not to the temples. Because your facial features are so balanced, there's no need to apply the blush lower on your face; doing so would make your jaw look heavier.

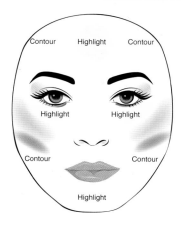

ROUND

Your goal for a round face is to reduce the roundness of the cheeks by cutting the cheeks in half—colorwise, of course.

Highlight: Apply highlight to the center of the face—the forehead, under the eyes, and the chin—to bring attention to these areas. Avoid highlight on the cheekbones, especially in the temple area; doing so will only make the area more pronounced.

Contour: Apply contour in the hollows of the cheeks. Add contour in a diagonal line to visually divide the cheeks in half, thus reducing the roundness of the cheeks.

Blush: Apply the desired cheek color in between the highlight and contour.

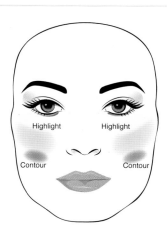

SQUARE

For the square face shape, you're basically doing the opposite of the round face shape—creating roundness instead of diminishing it. This softens an otherwise strong face shape.

Highlight: Apply highlight above the cheekbones on a diagonal to soften the strong lines of the face.

Contour: Apply contour to the hollows of the cheeks, creating a thin oval on the diagonal line. The slight oval creates roundness in the lower cheeks.

Blush: Apply blush in a circular motion from the temple down to the apples of the cheeks, almost like placing a check mark on the cheeks. Doing so further creates roundness in the cheeks.

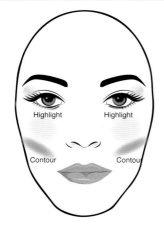

OBLONG (RECTANGLE)

The longest of the face shapes is the oblong face shape. The goal with this shape is to shorten the face while also creating softness in the cheek area similar to the square face shape.

Highlight: Apply highlight from the temple to under the eyes using a diagonal line to soften the face shape.

Contour: Apply contour to the diagonal line in the hollow part of the cheeks. Doing so gives the illusion of roundness.

Blush: Apply blush in a circular manner close to the apples of the cheeks to continue softening the facial features.

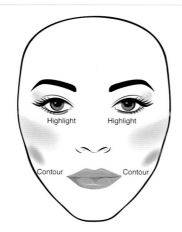

HEART

The heart face shape is wider at the top and narrow at the bottom. Your goal is to reduce some of the width at the top of the face to balance the narrow chin.

Highlight: Apply a slight horizontal highlight above the cheek-bones to focus attention on this area.

Contour: Apply contour just under the cheeks and blend downward to add a bit of fullness to the jawline.

Blush: Apply blush between the highlight and contour on a slight horizontal to give the illusion of less space between the eyes.

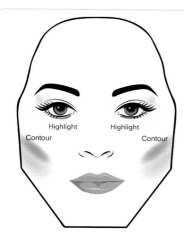

DIAMOND

The strongest feature on this face shape is the cheekbones. Therefore, you should make your prominent cheeks appear they are moving back into the face shape.

Highlight: Because the cheekbones are already prominent, keep your highlight under the eyes, sweeping it slightly up and out.

Contour: Apply contour such as a bronzer into the cheekbones to recede the cheeks into the face shape.

Blush: Apply blush just below contour to finish off your look.

More Secrets to Applying Blush!

- Most brushes that come with a blush are useless. Throw them out and invest in a blush brush that is slightly larger than the apples of your cheeks.
- Cream blush can be used on the lips for a complementary sheer and soft look.
- Powder blush should always be applied in one direction to avoid streaking.
- To find out the actual position of the apple of your cheek, look into the mirror, smile, and then sweep a blush brush upward in an arc from your cheekbone to your hairline.
- Some dark blush on the tip of your nose will make it look shorter. Blend the color in gently.
- For a natural look, use cream blush with cream foundation or powder blush with a powder foundation.

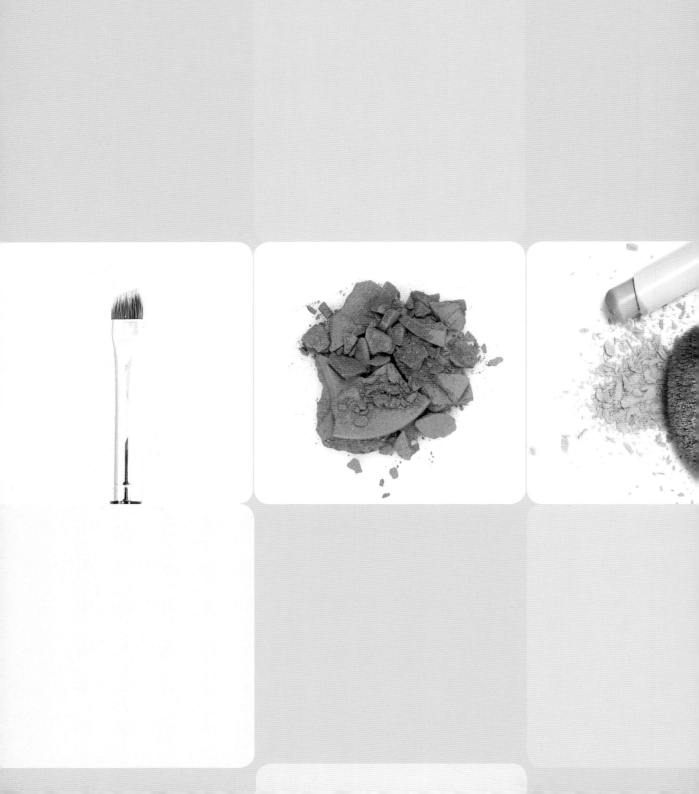

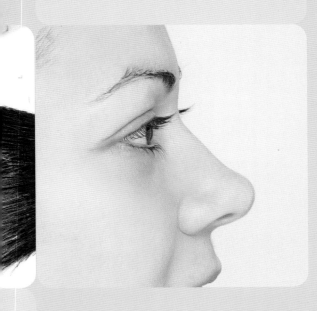

CHAPTER 8
NOSE

The nose is very important in facial symmetry because it's the center of the face. In art design, we use the term *emphasis*, which refers to where we want to draw a viewer's attention. Whatever the shape or size of your nose, you don't have to spend thousands of dollars visiting the plastic surgeon if you think it's too distracting. Using the magic of highlighting and contouring, you can alter your nose to the perfect proportion!

In this chapter, I address the different nose shapes and the corrective techniques you can use to make it complement your face.

WHAT YOU SHOULD KNOW ABOUT YOUR NOSE

The nose is divided into four main areas: the bridge, sidewalls, tip, and nostrils.

When it comes to creating the most balanced look to your face, your nose should be in proportion to the rest of your face. What does that involve? The following are guidelines to the ideal length and width of your nose.

Length of the nose: The center of the eyebrows to the tip of the nose should be equal to the distance from the hairline to the brow and the tip of the nose to the chin.

Width of the nose: The nostrils should be directly below the tear ducts of the eyes.

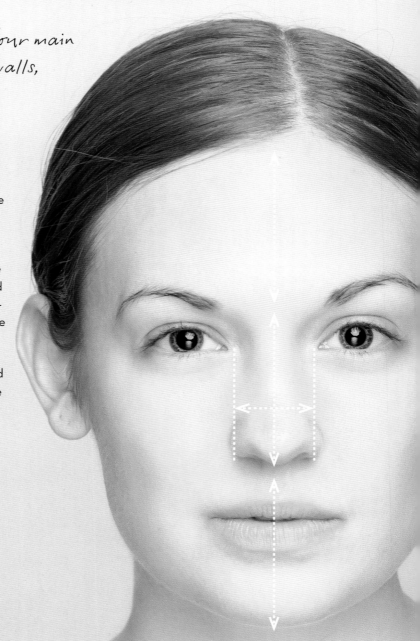

NOSE HIGHLIGHT AND CONTOUR SHADES AND TOOLS

You can correct a wide, thin, or even crooked nose with highlight and contour.

Let's first go over what you need to accomplish this.

Contour: Use a powder or cream color that's a half to full shade darker than your natural skin or foundation color.

Highlight: Use a powder or cream color that's a half to full shade lighter than your natural skin or foundation color.

Angle brush or small shadow brush: An angle brush will give a more precise line down the bridge of your nose, while a small shadow brush will create a softer line down it. Additionally, you can use the small shadow brush to blend the contour.

Disposable makeup sponge or beauty sponge: You can use a damp disposable makeup sponge or the smallest point of a damp beauty sponge to blend nose highlight and contour.

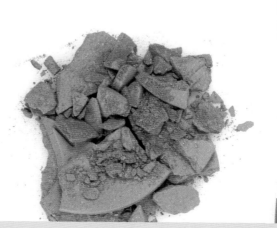

HIGHLIGHTING AND CONTOURING YOUR NOSE BY NOSE SHAPE

Whether your nose is too long for your face or you want to "fix" a crooked nose, I can help!

Highlighting and contouring using an angle brush, a small eye shadow brush, and/or a sponge can address various nose shapes and concerns. Remember, these corrections should be subtle, especially for daytime makeup. The following addresses how to slim down a wide nose, widen a thin nose, shorten a long nose, lengthen a short nose, and straighten a crooked nose. Natural noses don't need any highlighting or contouring.

WIDE

When you have a wide nose, the goal is to reduce the appearance of the width of the nose. This is achieved by reducing the sidewalls and emphasizing the center of the nose.

Highlight: Apply highlight straight down the bridge at the width and length you would like your nose to be. This placement helps the nose appear thinner.

Contour: Apply a shadow or darker foundation to the sides of the nose, using the side of your tool to create a line down each side of the highlight. Blend contour down the sidewalls to complete the look.

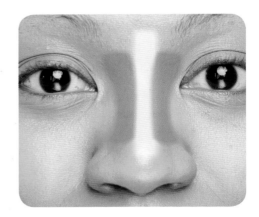

Highlighting Caution

Be careful not to make the highlight line on your nose's bridge too thin. You don't want to your nose to look like a toothpick!

THIN

If you have a thin nose, you should use your makeup to create the appearance of more width. Widening highlight past the sidewalls achieves this look.

Highlight: Apply highlight just past the bridge of the nose.

Contour: Apply shadow, darker foundation, or bronzer to the nose, using the side of the brush to create a line down each side of the highlight. These lines should run past the bridge into the sidewalls. Drag contour down the sidewalls to finish.

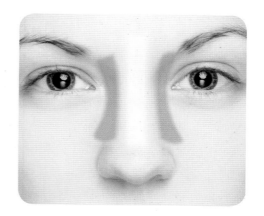

LONG

With long noses, reducing the appearance of the length is the primary goal. This is achieved by stopping highlight at the desired length of the nose.

Highlight: Starting at the top of the bridge, pull highlight down the bridge of the nose. Do not bring any highlight into the tip of the nose, as doing so will visually stop the eye from traveling downward.

Contour: Apply contour just under the tip of the nose, being careful not to blend it into the tip too much. This avoids making your nose look dirty from contour.

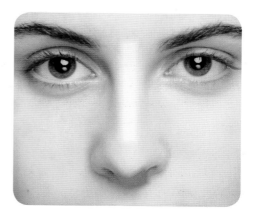

HIGHLIGHTING AND CONTOURING YOUR NOSE BY NOSE SHAPE

SHORT

For a short nose, it's important to lengthen the appearance of it. In this case, highlight is pulled to the tip of the nose and contour extends into the nostrils.

Highlight: Starting at the top of the bridge, drag highlight to the tip of the nose to visually create length.

Contour: Apply contour to the sides of the nose. Bring contour all the way down the nose to the nose's tip (following the highlight) to finish.

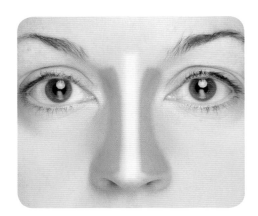

CROOKED

Even if your nose is crooked, highlight and contour can "fix" it, giving the appearance of a straight nose.

Highlight: Imagine where the line of a straight nose should be on your crooked nose. Drag highlight straight down to the tip of the nose following this imaginary line. It's okay if you overlap the sidewalls; highlight corrects the shadows that define a crooked nose.

Contour: Using your applied highlight line as a guide, apply contour on either side of this new line. Blend contour down the sidewalls to finish.

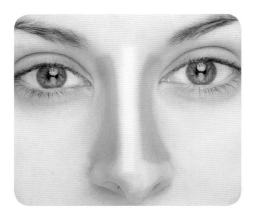

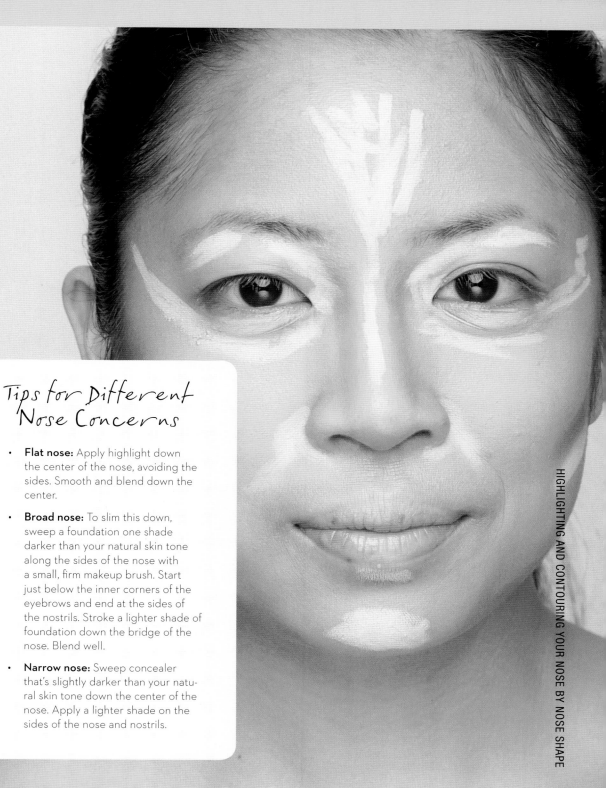

Tips for Different Nose Concerns

- **Flat nose:** Apply highlight down the center of the nose, avoiding the sides. Smooth and blend down the center.

- **Broad nose:** To slim this down, sweep a foundation one shade darker than your natural skin tone along the sides of the nose with a small, firm makeup brush. Start just below the inner corners of the eyebrows and end at the sides of the nostrils. Stroke a lighter shade of foundation down the bridge of the nose. Blend well.

- **Narrow nose:** Sweep concealer that's slightly darker than your natural skin tone down the center of the nose. Apply a lighter shade on the sides of the nose and nostrils.

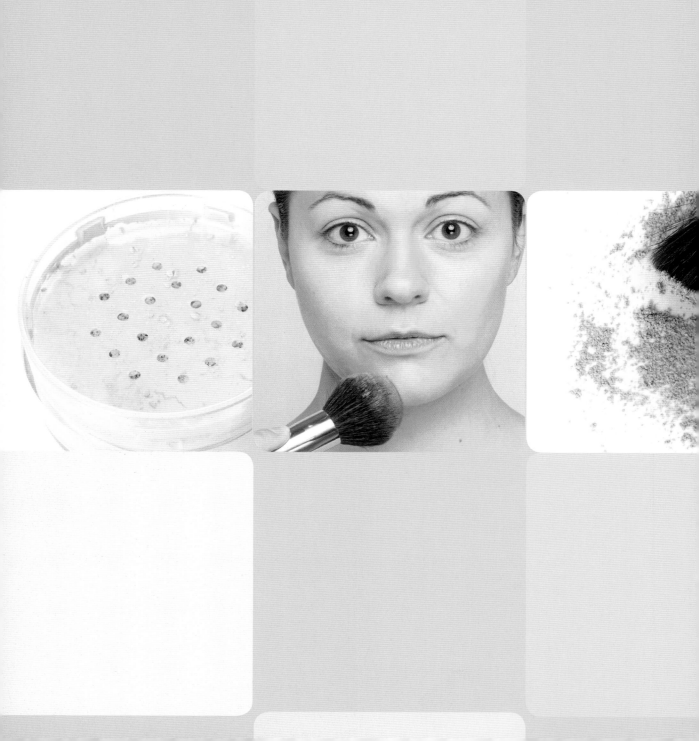

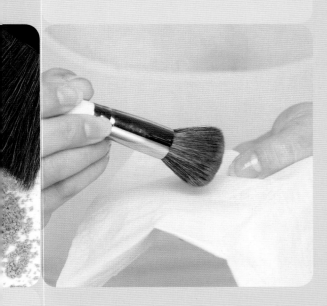

CHAPTER 9
SETTING POWDER

After applying concealer and foundation and contouring your face, cheeks, and nose, it's time to apply setting powder. Setting powder is used to reduce sweat on your face, set cream foundation, and blend your highlight and contour—in other words, it "sets" your face makeup.

In this chapter, I take you through the types of setting powder available, what you can use to put it on, and the best way to apply it.

TYPES OF SETTING POWDER

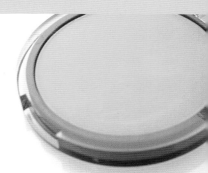

There are several types of setting powders that work well on their own on normal to oily skin types, with the exception of mineral powder, which works well for all skin types.

The following are the basic types available, as well as their best features.

Pressed powder: This comes in a compact and is great for absorbing oily skin, reducing shine, and setting your foundation.

Loose powder: This is similar to pressed powder, but it's more finely milled. This means you can layer the loose powder for better coverage. Loose powder typically comes in a shaker container; holes in the container's top assist in controlling the amount of product you are using and help to contain spillage.

Translucent powder: This is a setting powder that does not contain pigment, so you can set your foundation without competing with the foundation's base color. Translucent powder works on any skin color.

Tinted setting powder: This is tinted in shades that complement various skin colors, adding a little color when you are not using a foundation. In addition, it is great in helping blend corrective makeup. I personally use tinted setting powder on my clients to blend out the highlights and contouring I create in a makeup application.

Mineral powder: This powder absorbs excess oil and reduces shine. Because mineral makeup is tinted and creates a glowing look, I often use it as a setting powder. The trick is to use a foundation brush versus a kabuki brush. Foundation brushes have fewer bristles, which leave less powder on the skin than a kabuki brush.

Avoiding Pressed Powder Breakage

Having trouble with your pressed powder staying together? Place a cotton ball or round cotton pad in your powder compact to keep your pressed powder from breaking in your purse or cosmetic bag.

POWDER APPLICATION TOOLS

Setting powder can be applied with a powder puff, a powder brush, or even a kabuki brush. It all depends on how heavily you want the powder to go on and how you'd like to blend.

Powder puff: A powder puff typically comes with pressed or loose powder. It's made of a soft material that's used to press powder into the skin. You can also use the powder puff to blend contours and highlights into the skin after you put on your setting powder. Because reusing a powder puff will cause oil and debris to move from the face to the compact, you might consider investing in a powder puff you can launder.

Powder brush: The largest of the brushes, a powder brush has longer hairs to dust the setting powder onto your skin. It is easier to clean than a powder puff and can be used with all setting powder products. However, it is especially effective with loose powder because the longer and less dense brush offers a lighter application.

Kabuki brush: Because of its short, dense hairs, you have the option of using this brush to blend your makeup with the setting powder.

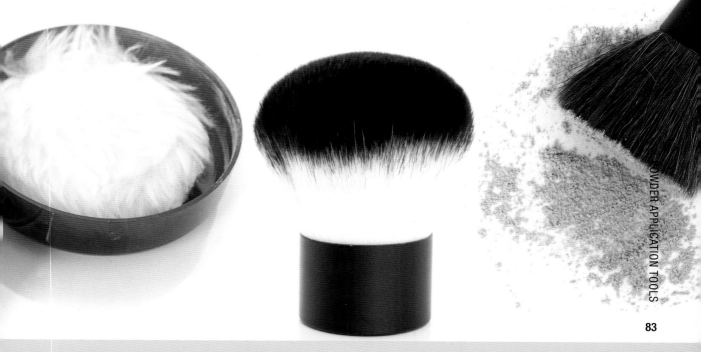

APPLYING SETTING POWDER

Setting powder has many functions, such as setting makeup so it doesn't come off and blending your highlight and contour into your skin.

It is not about providing more coverage like a foundation or concealer; the setting powder should simply give your face a softer look and help the foundation and concealer to stay on longer.

BASIC APPLICATION

The following is a basic application for setting powder, which mirrors foundation application. Use a light hand so as to not remove the foundation and concealer.

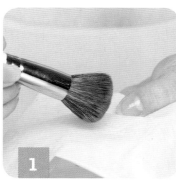

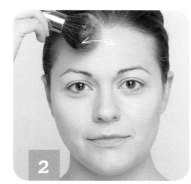

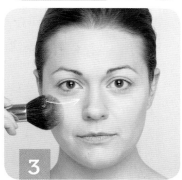

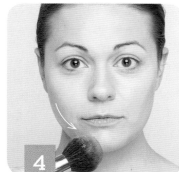

1. Tap any excess powder off of the powder brush.

2. Apply the setting powder starting at the forehead and brushing back and forth horizontally.

3. Move your brush down the side of the nose and horizontally under the eyes.

4. Brush your brush horizontally over the cheek down to the chin. Repeat on the opposite side.

BLENDING YOUR HIGHLIGHT AND CONTOUR

You have the option of using tinted or translucent setting powder to blend your highlight and contour so they don't sit on top of your foundation and concealer. Unlike the basic application, you are pressing rather than brushing the powder into the skin to adequately blend in the highlight and contour.

BEFORE

AFTER

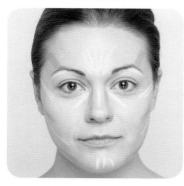
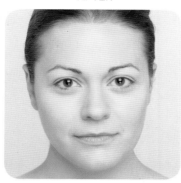

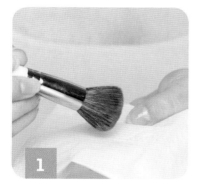
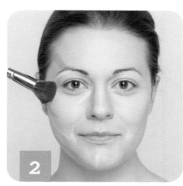

Using a Hydrating Mist

If you want your makeup to last longer, spray a hydrating mist after you apply your setting powder. The water more fully sets the powder into your skin.

1. Press your powder puff or kabuki brush into the setting powder.

2. Press your powder into the skin; do not brush back and forth. You are essentially pushing the highlight and contour color into the foundation, otherwise known as blending your makeup.

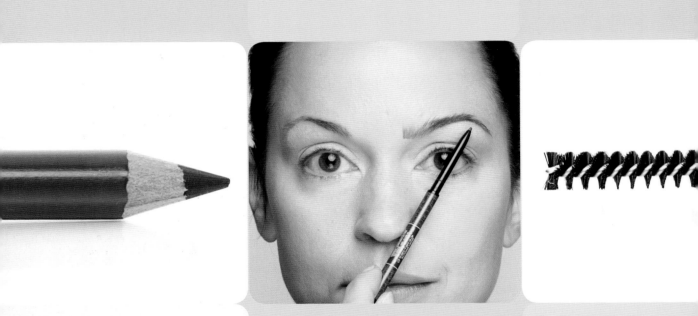

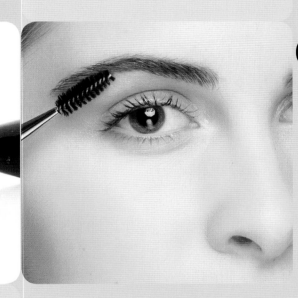

CHAPTER 10
EYEBROWS

If the eyes are the windows to the soul, the eyebrows are the valance to those windows! You can do a beautiful eye shadow application; however, the look will fall short if your eyebrows are not shaped and shaded correctly. This makes it critical to have your eyebrows looking their best.

This chapter focuses on eyebrows for your face shape, brow shaping techniques, and how to fill in your brows.

THE PERFECT EYEBROW

Before I get into grooming and shaping your eyebrows, let's talk about where your eyebrow should start, angle, and end.

Using a makeup brush, we're going to identify these three points of the perfect eyebrow.

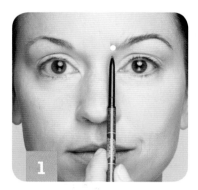 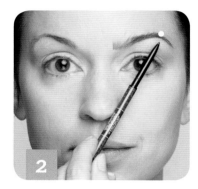 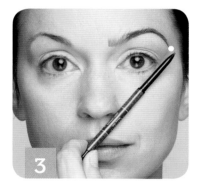

1. Place your makeup brush vertical with the side of your nose. This is where your eyebrow should begin.

2. Pivot your brush off your nose until it crosses your pupil. This will be the highest point of your arch. Your brow should arch on an angle to the right or left of your pupil—not above it!

3. Place your makeup brush on an angle from your nose to the outside corner of your eye. This is where your brow should end.

Shaping Overtweezed Brows

Have you overtweezed your eyebrows to the point you can no longer see their shape? I suggest drawing your "future" eyebrow over your current brow using an eye pencil or an eye shadow with an angle brush. You can even take a picture if you need to remember the shape. Once that's done, tweeze around the drawn eyebrow. It may take weeks to see the desired brow shape, but it's worth the wait!

EYEBROW TYPES

You may not realize it, but the shape of your eyebrows can be a key piece of a successful makeup.

There are five different eyebrow shapes you can have or sculpt—round, angled, soft angled, curved, and flat.

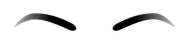

ROUND

A round eyebrow is an even curve without points.

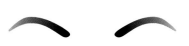

ANGLED

An angled eyebrow comes to a stronger peak before sloping downward. It's a stronger eyebrow than the traditional round shape.

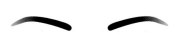

SOFT ANGLED

A soft-angled eyebrow is similar to an angled one. However, instead of coming to a strong point, it curves slightly at its peak.

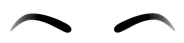

CURVED

A curved eyebrow has two curves—a smaller upside-down U, followed by a larger curve over the brow bone.

FLAT

A flat eyebrow does not have a strong peak. The brow is more horizontal, with a subtle slope at the end.

THE BEST EYEBROWS FOR EACH FACE SHAPE

My favorite moment as a makeup artist is reshaping my clients' brows.

It frames their eye makeup, balances their face shape, and adds that perfect pop of drama. I'd like to show you how to attain your perfect face shape with a suitable eyebrow shape.

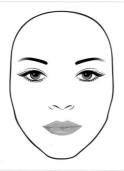

OVAL

While any eyebrow shape can work, soft-angled brows are the most attractive on this versatile face shape. Soft-angled brows complement the natural curve of an oval face.

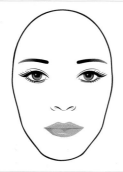

OBLONG (RECTANGLE)

Flat brows work best on the oblong face shape. This is because a long face needs more balance than any other shape, which thick, straight brows like the flat shape can provide. These brows are also good at not accentuating the length of it, unlike arched brows.

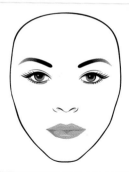

HEART

People with heart-shaped faces should ideally have rounded or curved brows. These brows help balance the pointy chin. Stay away from flat brows, which tend to overaccentuate the chin instead.

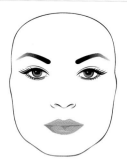

SQUARE

Curved or angled brows are recommended for a square-shaped face, which needs slimming for the four corners. Both brow types soften and balance the symmetry of this face shape. Stay away from an overly arched brow shape, as it can create an exaggerated jawline.

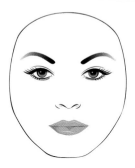

ROUND

Round faces look good with angled or soft-angled brows. Either brow can add length and strength to the face shape. Having the arch of the brows taper to a sharp point makes the cheekbones appear higher and the jawline look more distinct, for an overall elongating effect.

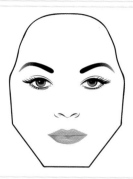

DIAMOND

A diamond face shape requires brows that balance the strong cheekbones. Therefore, anyone with this face shape should go with round, curved, or angled brows to narrow it.

BROW SHAPING

The perfect brow shape does wonders for your face.

Now that you know what brow works best with your features, it's time to look at how to shape your brows. While you're free to seek the help of a professional for this, there are a couple quick-and-easy ways you can shape your brows from the comfort of your own home: tweezing and waxing.

Tweezing: Using tweezers, a slender metal tool with a pointed or flat end, you pluck one hair at a time until you create the shape you desire. Be careful not to overpluck your eyebrows, or you'll end up having to shade them in.

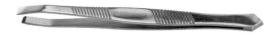

Waxing: This requires a pot of heated wax and a wooden spatula. The spatula is dipped into heated wax, and then the wax is applied to the area on the brow where you'd like to remove hair. After a few moments, you pull it off in the direction of the hair growth. There are two kinds of wax used in this technique: soft and hard wax.

Soft wax is the consistency of honey. When heated, it can be applied with a wooden spatula and removed with a cloth strip. It removes the hair quickly. While redness often follows a soft wax, it should go away within an hour. You can apply aloe afterward to reduce any redness and irritation.

Hard wax is a great option for those with sensitive skin or on acne medication, which can make the skin thin and easily irritated. This technique does not require a cloth for removal. The wax dries, holding the hair in the product. You then simply pull the hard wax off, removing the hairs with it.

Threading

Originating from India, threading is a fast and inexpensive brow-shaping technique that has become very popular internationally. In threading, a thin cotton thread is doubled, twisted, and then rolled across areas where the hair needs to be removed. This motion pulls the hair out at the follicle, one hair at a time.

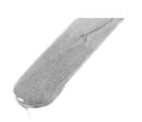

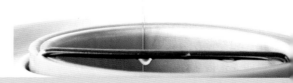

Waxing at Home

Not getting the eyebrow waxing results you want? Follow these steps using the indicated products (which you can find at beauty supply stores or online), and you'll get perfectly waxed eyebrows every time!

Small cosmetic scissors

Prewax cleanser

Baby powder

Wax applicator (such as a wooden spatula)

Heated soft wax

Pellon or muslin cloth strips

Baby oil or wax remover

Aloe vera

1. Before waxing, pull your hair back from your face and shape your eyebrows to your desired shape. If necessary, trim your eyebrows with small cosmetic scissors.

2. Apply prewax cleanser to your eyebrows; this will help you avoid any infection.

3. Dab baby powder on your eyebrows. This acts as a barrier between the wax and your skin.

4. Using your eyebrow wax applicator, apply wax in the direction your eyebrows grow, making sure all the eyebrows you want to remove have wax. Remember, only apply it to the hairs you want to remove.

5. Cover your eyebrow with pellon or muslin cloth strip in the direction of your eyebrow growth; a part of the strip should be free of hair for removal. Firmly press the strip in the direction your eyebrow grows several times to ensure it has been attached to the hairs, and let it cool slightly.

6. Grasp the part of the cloth strip extended beyond the eyebrow and, holding your eyebrow skin taut with your other hand, remove the strip with one quick pull in the opposite direction of the hair growth (*not* upward). If any hairs are remaining, put the strip back on and pull it off again.

7. Clean any remaining wax off your skin using baby oil or a wax remover.

8. Finish by applying aloe vera to reduce redness.

FILLING IN BROWS

Think of this step as creating a shadow behind the brows.

To do this, use a shade lighter than the brow color and fill in. If your eyebrow is very blonde, choose a color a shade or two darker than your brow. While many companies have developed products for shading your eyebrows, it's really quite simple to do yourself. Let's take a look.

TOOLS FOR FILLING IN

The following are tools you can use when shaping your brows. Pencils are a great tool when you need to lengthen or fill in a weak brow, while eye shadows are used to add more color and fullness to a brow. You can use each separately or together, depending on your need.

Eyebrow pencil: You can use the point of an eyebrow pencil to lightly draw in hairs for a natural look, or shade in the brows for a more dramatic look. There are five shades typically used to fill; each is matched to a particular hair color:

> **Taupe:** Blonde and red hair
>
> **Light brown:** Dark blonde and light brown hair
>
> **Medium brown:** Light to medium brown hair
>
> **Dark brown:** Medium to dark brown hair
>
> **Black:** Black hair and dark skin

Eye shadow: You can use a matte eye shadow with an angle brush to fill in and shape your brows. Again, I suggest you use the shade that corresponds with your hair color:

> **Taupe:** Blonde hair
>
> **Light brown:** Light to medium brown hair
>
> **Dark brown:** Dark brown hair
>
> **Black:** Black hair

BASIC BROW FILLING

Ultimately, your goal is to give the illusion of a fuller natural brow. The following walks you step by step through how to do this. Refer back to "The Perfect Eyebrow" if necessary for a refresher on the three points of the brow.

1. Point 1 should be the darkest and fullest area of the eyebrow. Use the tip of your pencil and begin by drawing a line vertical to the nose.

2. Lightly draw the bottom line of the brow from the starting point, over the arch, and down to point 3.

3. Lightly create a parallel line at the top of the brow you are creating.

4. Use a lighter touch as you move from point 2 to point 3 to give a softer finish to the brow. The brow should become thinner as you get to point 3.

5. Lightly fill in between the two lines. Remember, the brow should be darker between points 1 and 2 and begin to become lighter as you move toward point 3.

6. If you'd like, you can use a disposable mascara wand to brush over the eyebrow you created. The mascara wand softens the lines and blends them into your natural eyebrows.

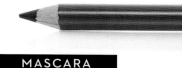

What You Need

EYEBROW PENCIL

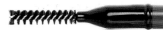

MASCARA WAND

Creating an Eyelift

For an instant eyelift, apply soft white eye shadow above your eyebrow and soft pink eye shadow in below the arch of your eyebrow. This will define and elevate it.

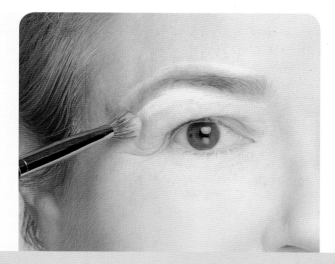

Creating a Brow Stencil

To simplify fill in your eyebrows, you can create a brow stencil.

Vellum paper

Craft razor

Cutting mat

Number-2 pencil

Hold the vellum paper to your eyebrow and lightly trace your eyebrow, using the eyebrow shape as a guide.

Choose the eyebrow shape you would like to create: round, angled, soft angled, curved, or flat. Sketch the shape over the brow you traced on the vellum paper. Erase the parts of the old brow you don't want and then, using the craft razor, cut the remaining brow shape out of the vellum. Use the point of your craft razor to cut out the inside of the stencil.

If you would like to have a stencil for each brow, turn the stencil upside down and trace a mirror image of the brow. Using the craft razor, cut out the second brow stencil. Label one stencil R (right) and the other L (left).

Place the stencil over your eyebrow and color it in with the appropriate eyebrow pencil or matte eye shadow. If you are using only one stencil, turn the stencil over and place it on the opposite brow; otherwise, use the second stencil.

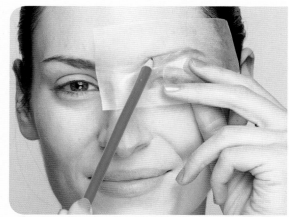

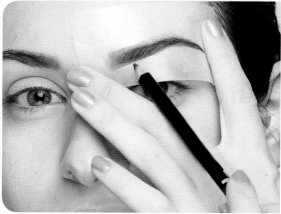

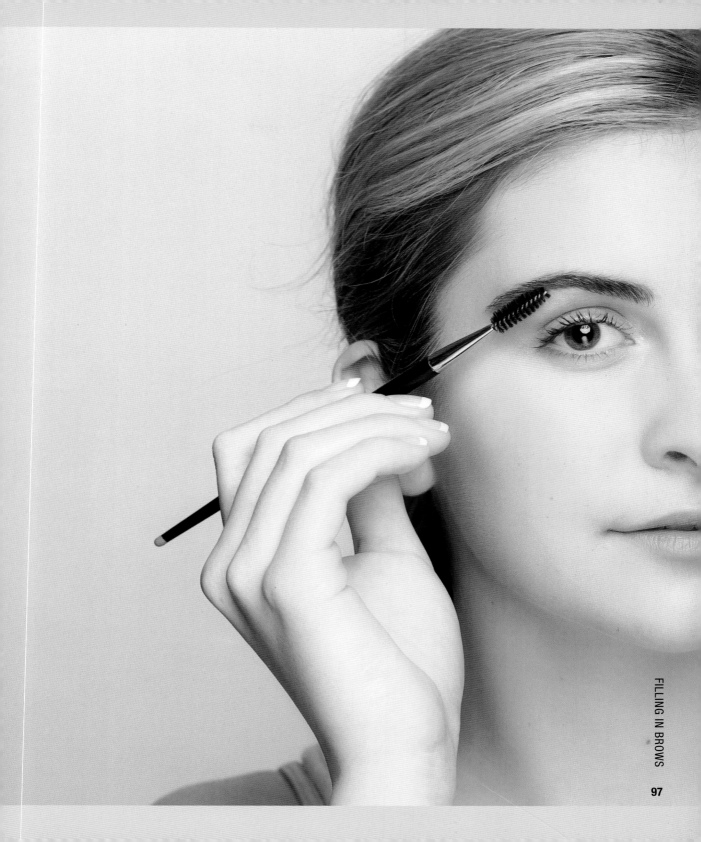

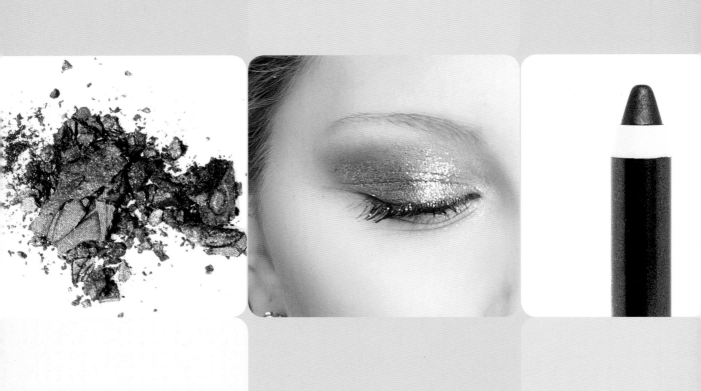

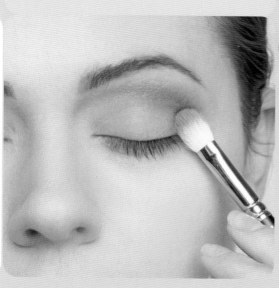

CHAPTER 11
EYE SHADOW

With entire stores designated just to eye shadow
options, choosing the right texture, hue, and brand
can seem incredibly intimidating. Don't allow the vast
variety to scare you though—embrace it!

In this chapter, I help you choose the appropriate
eye shadow products and color. I also give you some
application tips so you can make your eyes look their
most dazzling.

TYPES OF EYE SHADOWS

There are thousands of eye shadow pigments (or colors).

These shadows come in the following forms: pressed powder, loose powder, cream, and mineral.

Pressed powder: Eye shadow in pressed form comes in a compact, which makes it easy to carry. You can apply pressed powder with a brush, a sponge applicator, or an applicator supplied with the shadow.

Loose powder: Eye shadow in loose form comes in a shaker. This type of eye shadow is applied with brush. For a bolder eye look, use loose powder for a stronger application of pigment.

Cream: This comes in a variety of colors and provides more coverage due to its thicker consistency. However, because it is a cream, it can easily crease; therefore, I don't recommend cream shadow for mature eyes.

Mineral: This eye shadow is great alternative to the other shadow types. It comes in beautiful colors and is great for sensitive skin, as it doesn't irritate.

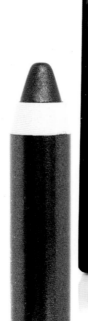
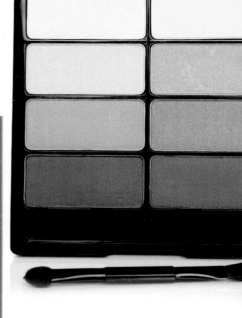

Setting Your Eye Shadow

For longer wear, use cream shadow as a primer for a pressed or loose eye shadow in the same color. You can then apply the powder shadow to set the cream.

EYE SHADOW FINISHES

Another difference between eye shadows is the type of finish they have: sheer, matte, shimmer, metallic, or glitter.

Sheer: These eye shadows have a light pigment. They provide a hint of color and are great to use for everyday natural looks.

Matte: Shadows that do not have a shine or reflection of light are referred to as having a matte finish. Matte shadows are often beautiful, silky colors that are used for natural looks. They are great for mature eyes, since they will not highlight the fine lines associated with aging.

Shimmer: These types of eye shadow contain light-reflecting materials that provide their shimmer finish, giving depth and interest to the colors. In addition, you can easily blend shades in this finish to create a striking look.

Metallic: These eye shadows are similar to a shimmer shadow in terms of their finish. They typically come in shades the color of metal (gold, silver, copper, and black). Metallic finishes create a dramatic evening look and are great on darker skin.

Glitter: Cosmetic glitter is ground a bit finer than craft glitter and gives a sparkle to eye shadows. Glitter finish creates a theatrical eye effect and is typically worn by teenage girls. Because glitter is loose and can shed easily, it should be the last thing you apply when doing your makeup.

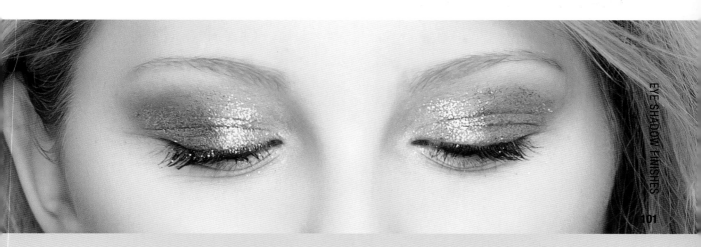

CHOOSING AN EYE SHADOW COLOR

You may be wondering, "How do I choose a color that looks best on me?"

Any good makeup artist will tell you it's important to first have an understanding of the color wheel. So before you pick out eye shadow, let's review the color wheel and the relationship between primary, secondary, and tertiary colors.

All colors derive from the *primary colors:* red, yellow, and blue. Primary colors cannot be mixed or formed by another color. *Secondary colors* are a combination of two primary colors, which result in orange, green, and violet, depending on the colors combined. *Tertiary colors* are a combination of a primary and a secondary color. For example, red-orange, red-violet, yellow-orange, yellow-green, blue-violet, and blue-green are tertiary colors.

All colors have complementary colors, which are colors that are opposite each other on the color wheel. When combined in the right proportions, these pairs will create white or black. Here are some common examples:

- Red is complementary to the color green.

- Blue is complementary to the color orange.

- Yellow is complementary to the color violet.

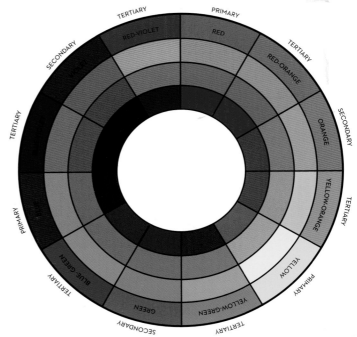

Now that you understand the color wheel, a good rule of thumb to follow is to use your eye color to help indicate the appropriate color choice. Here are the eye shadow shades I recommend based on eye color.

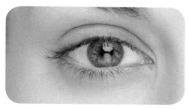

Blue eyes: The complementary color to blue is orange. Therefore, look for colors that have shades of orange, such as gold, copper, apricot, and peach.

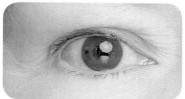

Green eyes: The complementary color to green is red. So look for eye shadow in shades of red, such as plum and wine.

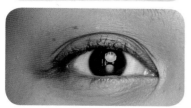

Brown eyes: Brown is a neutral color, so any eye shadow color will work with it. Typically, blue and purple are standout colors for brown eyes.

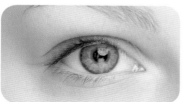

Hazel eyes: Women with hazel eyes are able to enjoy a wide spectrum of shadow shades due to the flecked hues they possess. This eye color can handle many shades of eye makeup. However, blue is one exception; this color can make the eyes look grayish.

Salvaging Your Eye Shadow

Did you drop your eye shadow? No problem! Here are a couple ways you can salvage it:

- If you want to still use it as shadow, add a few drops of rubbing alcohol to the broken shadow. You can then pat it back together with a quarter, thus reshaping and remixing the shadow.

- For something different, take the eye shadow and mix it with a clear nail polish. You have now created some great nail polish!

APPLYING EYE SHADOW 101

Once you've chosen the appropriate colors for your skin tone, eye color, and eye shadow design, it's time to apply them.

Basic shadow placement begins with putting on three eye shadow colors: light, medium, and dark. You then proceed to blend the eye shadow colors into one another; this softens the lines between colors and any harsh lines. For the best outcome, the entire lid should be covered in makeup. Leaving any part of the lid exposed can weaken the overall look.

What You Need

EYE SHADOW BRUSH

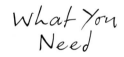

LIGHT EYE SHADOW

DARK EYE SHADOW

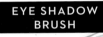

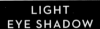

MEDIUM EYE SHADOW

1. Apply the medium eye shadow color on your eyelid. This color is typically the predominant color (for example, gold) and is the statement color in the palette.

2. Apply the dark eye shadow color in the crease of your eye; these are usually made up of shades of brown or black. This is a form of contouring that creates definition for the eye.

3. Apply the light eye shadow color from the crease to just under the eyebrow and from the brow bone into the tear duct. This is a white, ivory, or cream color used to highlight the eye.

4. Using your eye shadow brush, blend the darkest color just into the highlight color, moving back and forth like a windshield wiper. Repeat the blending into the medium eye shadow color. Remember to only blend where a color meets a color; pulling a color completely into another will make the application appear sloppy and muddy.

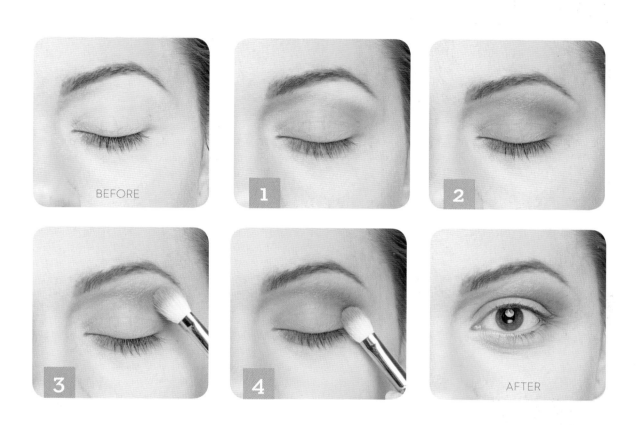

BEFORE

1

2

3

4

AFTER

Making Colors Pop

Want to make colored eye shadows pop? First, apply a white eye cream to the eyelid, and then dab your favorite eye shadow color on top. The white eye cream will intensify the colored eye shadow.

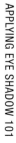

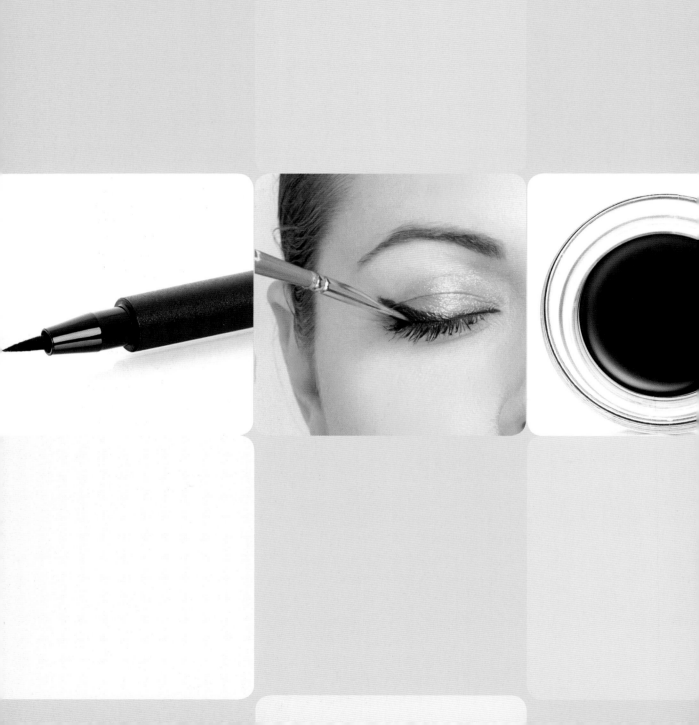

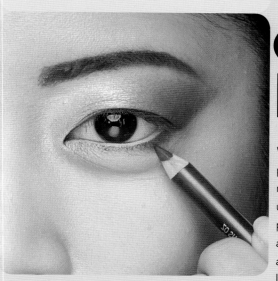

CHAPTER 12
EYELINER

When I was little, I loved to outline my coloring book pictures in black because the effect made them look more polished. The same effect happens when you use eyeliner on your eyes. Eyeliner makes the eyes pop, creates a polished look, and grounds the makeup application. Of course, eyeliner is a privilege and not a right; it's about creating a dramatic outline without looking like you are stuck in the '80s.

In this chapter, I give you tips on eyeliner, from basic application to creating more dramatic looks.

TYPES OF EYELINER

Originally introduced by the Egyptians and gaining popularity in the 1920s, eyeliner has been used as a tool to accentuate the eyes.

While the first eyeliner was made from kohl (lead sulfite), manufacturers have since created eyeliner with much safer ingredients. You can find eyeliner in pencil, liquid, gel pot, and eye shadow form.

Pencil: Eyeliner pencils come in shades varying from white to black, are easy to apply, and are very affordable. You can find pencils in thin and jumbo sizes, depending on how thick you want the line to be. Typically, pencils and most gel pencils will require the use of a cosmetic pencil sharpener. Eyeliner pencils are particularly great to use for smoky eye applications because of the ease with which you can smudge them.

Liquid: This eyeliner goes on wet to dry and provides a stronger pigment of color than pencil. It also comes with a pen tip, which makes application much easier. Liquid liner requires a steady hand, but it's worth the effort when it comes to a clean look. Because liquid liner needs a moment to dry, I suggest keeping your eye closed for a few seconds; otherwise, smudging may occur.

Gel pot: Gel eyeliner comes in a small pot and is applied with an angle brush. This eyeliner has a stronger pigment like liquid eyeliner; however, you can smudge the product into place before it sets.

Eye shadow: You can also use eye shadow as a liner. In fact, I encourage you to use a matte eye shadow with a makeup brush prior to using a pencil or pen. If you are making a cat eye, you can lay down the eye shadow as a guide for your liner. Additionally, eye shadow as a liner is great for oily skin because it absorbs the oil, allowing the shadow to stay on the lid.

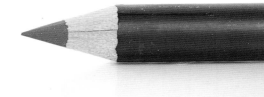

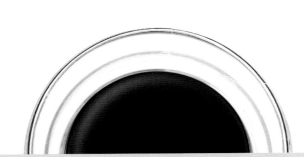

BASIC EYELINER APPLICATION

The following are the basic steps for applying eyeliner.

Remember, you should begin your eyeliner application only after you have completed applying your eye shadow.

1. Place your index finger at the crease of your eye and gently lift the eyelid. This is especially important if you have a heavy-fold eyelid or mature skin that has lost some of its elasticity.

2. Beginning at the last eyelash located closest to your tear duct, start drawing a line following the natural lash line. This may take a few strokes of the liner.

3. Stop at the end of your outer eye, being careful not to go past the eyelashes.

4. Repeat steps 2 and 3 on the lower lashline. For a natural look, start at the center of the eye and work to the outside corner. Blend at the center to create a soft line.

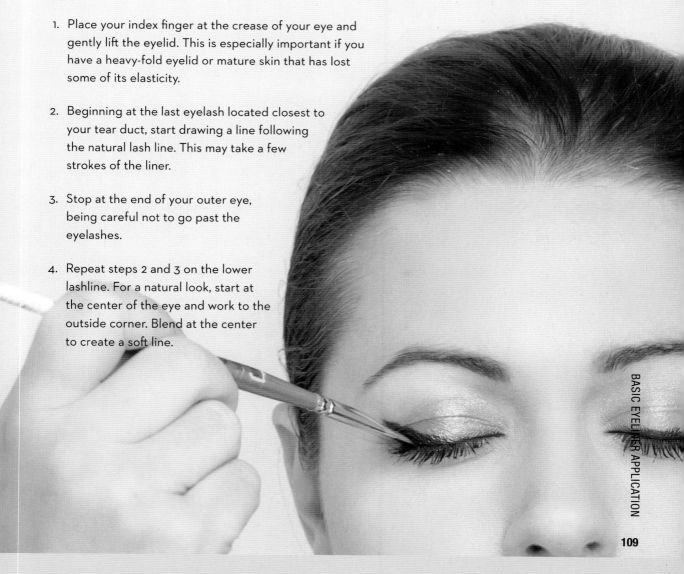

GOING BEYOND BASIC: EYELINER BY ERA

Looking for something beyond a basic line?

Different eras have provided looks that are fun and easy to copy. The following go through popular eyeliner in several decades, as well as the best eyeliner products to achieve them.

1920S

The 1920s was the time period that launched the smoky eye look of eyeliner with a coal effect. To create the 1920s smoky eye, take your eyeliner pencil or gel pot and follow the natural curve of the lash line, tracing all around the eye. Finally, smudge outside of the lower lash line; this creates a softer (smoky) effect with the liner.

1940S

The 1940s emphasized liner on top of the lid. To create this look, take your eyeliner pencil or liquid liner along the top lash line, following the curve of the eye with a thick line. On the bottom lash line, use an eye shadow or pencil to create a thin line, stopping before your tear duct.

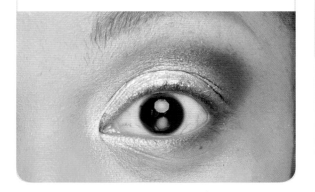

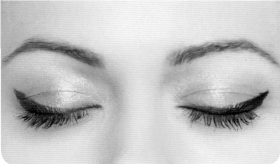

1950S AND 1960S

The cat eye trend began in the 1950s and became overexaggerated in the 1960s as outrageous fashion styles exploded. To create the bold eye, take a liquid or gel eyeliner and create a thick black line on the top lash line. When you approach the outer edge, swoop the liner upward.

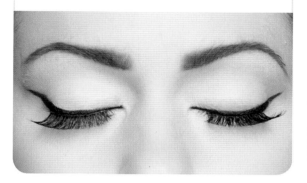

1970S

In the 1970s, eyeliner switched to a more natural look composed of browns and whites. To create this look, use a brown eyeliner and follow the natural curve of your lash line. Apply to the top only.

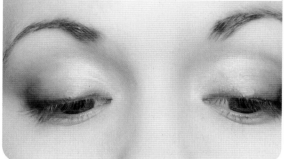

1980S

The style dictates you could use any-color eyeliner to complete your look, though black will be the most dramatic. To create this look, take any liner type and line completely around the entire eye and into the water line—in fact, the more severe and dramatic the eyeliner, the better.

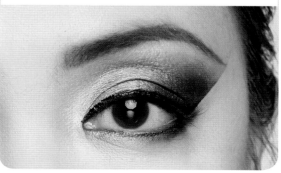

Polishing Your Eye Look

To give your makeup application a more polished look, take the primary eye shadow color you used on your eyelid and apply the same color along your bottom lash line using an angle brush. For example, if you used a turquoise eye shadow, use the same color in the tear duct area to marry the look together.

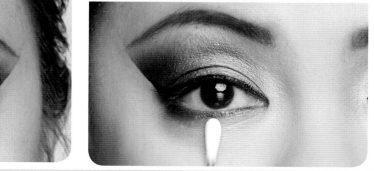

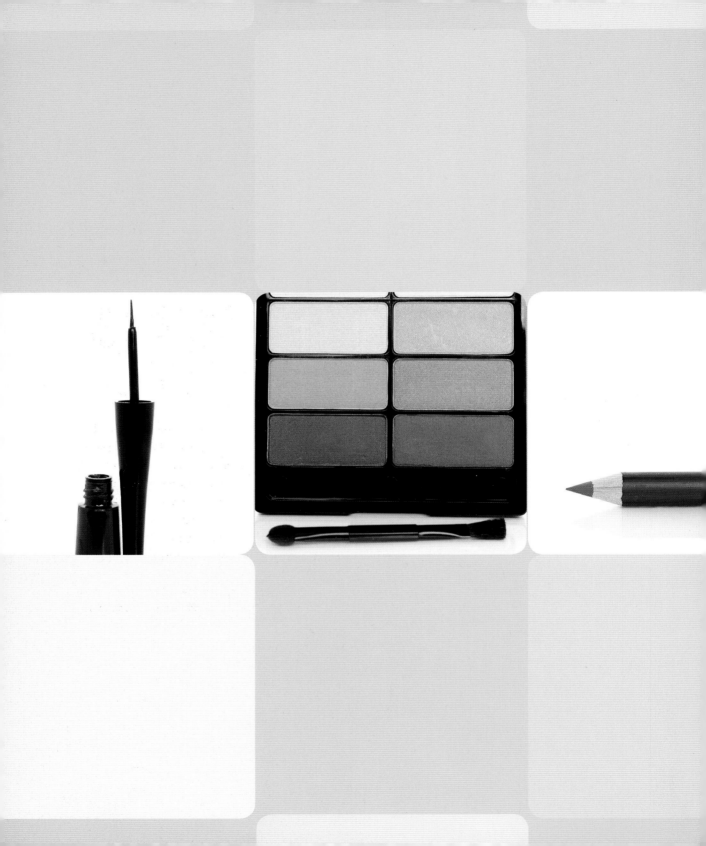

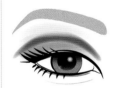
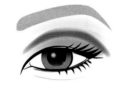

CHAPTER 13
FULL EYE

As is the case with face shapes, everyone is born with different eye shapes. The mistake made in eye makeup application is not understanding the shape of the eyes, especially if you see an application or technique applied to an eye different from your own. Therefore, now that I've gone through eye shadow and eye make-up, I'd like to show you how to bring those together to create the perfect look for your eye shape.

In this chapter, I give you highlighting and contouring techniques for different eye shapes using eye shadow and/or eyeliner.

PARTS OF THE EYE AND THEIR ROLE IN MAKEUP

With full eye makeup, the entire eye must be considered. Each part should be addressed during a makeup application.

- **Brow bone:** Found directly under the eyebrow, the highlight color is applied in this section.

- **Crease:** Found at the top of the lid and the beginning of the brow bone, it is the section where the skin rolls into the eye socket. Depending on the brow bone, the crease can be deep set to nonexistent.

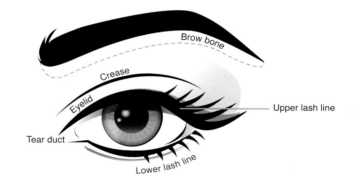

- **Eyelid:** The half-moon-shaped section of skin between the upper lash line and the crease, this is the primary space for eye shadow.

- **Upper lash line:** Found along the edge of the lid closest to the eye, this is where eyeliner, mascara, and false eyelashes are used.

- **Tear duct:** Also known as the *inner eye*, this is found at the corner of the eye closest to the nose. Liner and shadow can be placed in this section.

- **Lower lash line:** Found at the bottom of the eye, you use eyeliner and mascara in this section.

CORRECTING YOUR EYE SHAPE WITH FULL EYE MAKEUP

Now that you know the parts of the eye, it's time go over the 10 eye shapes—almond, wide set, close set, deep set, prominent, small, monolid, hooded, upturned, and downturned eye shapes—and how to correct them, if necessary, to create the perfect eye look.

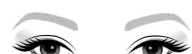

ALMOND (AVERAGE) EYES

This is the shape you want to replicate. The almond eye shape is the most balanced in width and height and has equal distance from the upper lash line to the crease and crease to the brow bone. If you have this eye shape, you will find it easy to create most eye makeup looks, no matter the technique.

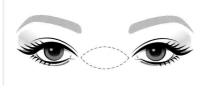

WIDE-SET EYES

Wide-set eyes are set more than an eye width apart. The goal of your eye makeup application should be to bring the eyes in toward the nose. Apply darker eye shadow colors in the corners of the eyes. This technique draws the eyes in toward the nose.

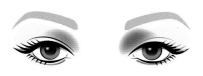

Eye shadow colors and placement can assist in bringing wide-set eyes inward. Use light eye shadow colors on the middle to outside eyes and darker eye shadow colors closer to the nose to draw focus inward. If you choose to wear dark eye shadows, do not apply past the end of the eyebrow; this accentuates the wideness of the eyes.

CLOSE-SET EYES

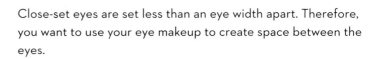

Close-set eyes are set less than an eye width apart. Therefore, you want to use your eye makeup to create space between the eyes.

The trick is to create more space between the bridge of the nose and the corners of the eyes. This is achieved by placing a light color, such as white, in the inside corners of the eyes.

DEEP-SET EYES

Deep-set eyes have protruding eye sockets. Because the eyes are set back farther into the eye socket, they create shadows. You want to reduce the shadows the eye sockets cast onto the eyelids.

Apply a light eye shadow on the eyelid, blending it into the eye socket, to lessen the shadows. To finish the application, apply a contour color in the creases and blend up and over the brow bones.

PROMINENT EYES

Prominent eye are large, round eyes where more of the white of the eyes can be seen. Your goal is to give the illusion the eyes are smaller than they seem.

Bring your darker eye shadows closer to the top lash lines. Follow up with a heavy, dark eyeliner on the top lash lines. Finish the application by adding your dark eyeliner into the water lines (the pink area behind your lower lashes) to give the illusion of smaller eyes.

SMALL EYES

Small eyes have little space between the lash lines, with very little of the whites of the eyes showing. Therefore, it's important to make the eyes look bigger and more pronounced.

Apply a white pencil along the lower lash lines. Apply eyeliner just below the white eyeliner. This technique gives the illusion of a larger eye shape.

MONOLID EYES

Monolid eyes have little to no crease in the eyelids and no brow bone. There is a fairly flat surface between the eyelid and the eyebrow. Monolid eyes provide a larger surface area to play with. Because there is an absence of a crease in the eyelids, you need to create that.

Apply the contour (darkest) shadow in a half-moon shape where you imagine a crease to be on each eye. Blend your medium shadow on the creases. Finally, apply the highlight eye shadow.

HOODED EYES

Hooded eyes have heavy folds of skin that hang over the eye sockets, which are more prominent in mature skin. The trick is to create a contour on the lids.

Sweep a matte contour color closest to the lash lines. Next, layer your medium eye shadow color above the contour, and blend highlight (light eye shadow) from the corner of the eyes upward into the brow bones. This reduces the weight in the eyelids.

Last, apply eyeliner into the upper lash lines. Remember, the lids are covering a lot of the eyes. Therefore, be careful not to make the liner too thick, as it will get lost in the folds.

UPTURNED EYES

Upturned eyes angle upward at the outer corners of the eyes. For example, most Disney princesses are drawn with upturned eyes! To minimize the amount of angle, imagine the eyelids are divided in half.

Apply a medium shadow from the center and blend downward toward the tear ducts. Apply the contour (darkest) color from the middle of the eyes toward the outer corners. Finish by blending the color in a "U" shape (not following the upward slope). This angles the eyes downward, creating the illusion that the eyes aren't so upturned.

DOWNTURNED EYES

Downturned eyes angle downward at the eyes' outer corners. To correct this, you want to give the eyes a lift.

Apply a medium shadow from the tear ducts to just past the middle of the eyes. Apply a contour color just past the middle of the eyes, sweeping it upward at the outer corners. This creates the lift you need.

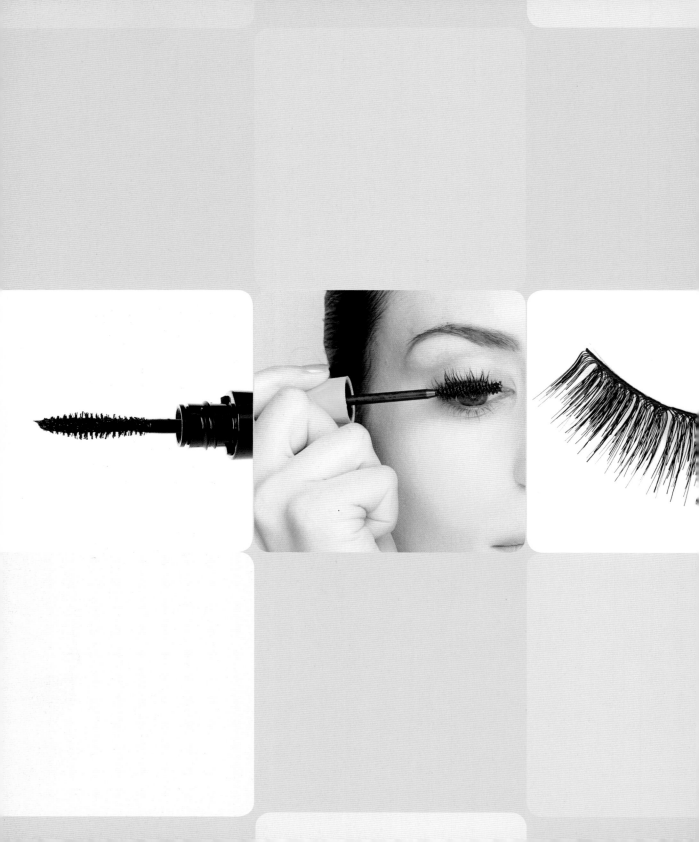

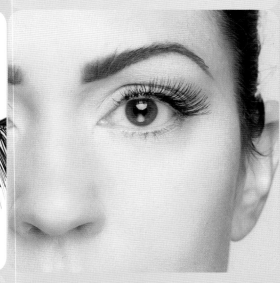

CHAPTER 14
EYELASHES

While eyelashes serve the important purpose of protecting your eyes from debris, I consider them ornamentation. They surround your eye like the fringe on a pillow; in the same way, they can complement your makeup application.

This chapter focuses on techniques to get the long, lush lashes you crave, including using mascara, curling wands, and false eyelashes.

TYPES OF MASCARA

Mascara is a cosmetic formulated with pigments, waxes, oils, and preservatives to darken and thicken the eyelashes.

Just like the hair on your head, eyelashes can be thin, brittle, and unruly. Therefore, different types of mascara have been designed to address these common issues.

Waterproof mascara: This type is formulated with mineral oils and waxes that enable it to stay on your eyelashes through tears, sweat, and water.

Volumizing mascara: The formula for this mascara contains silicone polymers and thickening agents, which give the illusion of thicker eyelashes.

Smudge-proof mascara: Formulated with a wax-oil base, this mascara is great for people who are very active and don't want to retouch their mascara during the day.

Curling mascara: This type is a bit thicker than regular mascara. It comes with a wand designed to curl the lashes.

Lengthening mascara: This mascara contains tiny synthetic fibers that cling to one another and to the lash, giving the appearance of longer lashes.

Lash-defining mascara: This provides a combination of volumizing, lengthening, and color to your eyelashes. Typically waterproof, it's considered an all-in-one mascara.

Primer mascara: This type is good if you wear makeup every day. It coats the lashes, protecting them from damage from daily mascara use. Primer also provides moisture to dry lashes and acts as a coat so your mascara goes on evenly.

Defining Your Lashes

Use an eyeliner pen to highlight your bottom eyelashes. While it takes some time, you can define each lash individually, making them stand out.

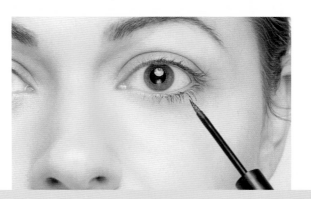

MASCARA COLORS

You can find mascara in a variety of colors, depending on your needs.

Black: Black mascara is great for a dramatic and bold look, and for use on darker skin tones.

Brown: Brown mascara is a bit softer than black mascara and works for natural daytime looks. It's a nice color choice for fair-complected skin types.

Fashion colors: This refers to colors beyond the typical black and brown, such as blue, yellow, and green. Fashion-color mascara helps enhance a dramatic, youthful look.

Clear: If you already have thick, full eyelashes and just want definition, try a clear mascara. It simply provides shine and separation for your lashes.

Mascara Application Tips

Do you ever put on your mascara to perfection, only to blink and have it stain and smudge? To avoid smudges on the skin beneath your lashes, lay a plastic spoon under your bottom lashes, and then apply your mascara. If you're looking to keep your upper lashes and eye makeup pristine, place an index card behind your top lashes when applying mascara.

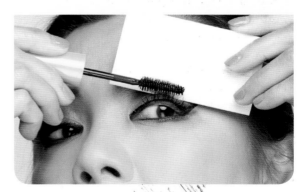

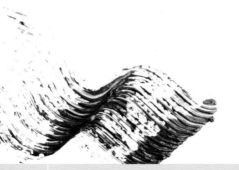

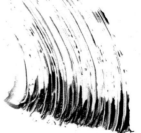

MASCARA WANDS

You might not realize it, but the proper mascara wand is just as important as the mascara itself.

The following are the different types of mascara wands you can find, as well as what specific lash issues they address.

Short wand: A mascara wand with short bristles is great for short eyelashes.

Long wand: This type of wand has evenly spaced bristles that are ideal for lengthening your lashes.

Round wand: A round wand with dense bristles can help you achieve volume in your lashes.

Spherical brush wand: This type of wand, with bristles on a sphere, is designed for individual eyelash application. While using this is more time consuming, you'll end up with well-defined lashes.

Curved wand: This wand has evenly spaced bristles that lift and curl your eyelashes.

Cleaning Off Excess Mascara

Do you always have too much product on your mascara wand? Wipe a little off on a tissue before applying. Pay close attention to the end of the wand, where product tends to gather and clump.

Recycling Your Wands

Looking to save some money? Keep your expensive and favorite wands from discarded mascaras, clean them off, and use them in less-expensive mascaras for better application.

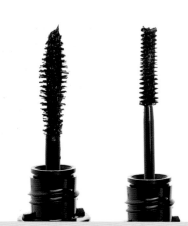

BASIC MASCARA APPLICATION

Applying mascara does not have to be difficult.

The basic rule of thumb is to apply to your top lashes only, unless you want your eyes to look more open. The following walks you through how to get the best mascara coverage for your lashes.

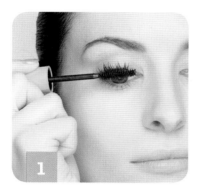
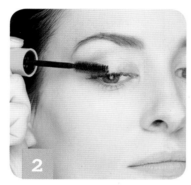
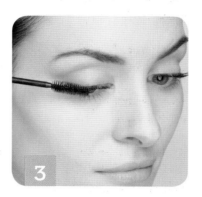

1. Place the mascara wand deep into the base of the lashes, wiggling it in left to right. You want to have good coverage near the roots, as it is mascara in that area—not the tips—that gives the illusion of length.

2. Pull the wand up and through the lashes, wiggling as you go. This wiggling helps separate the lashes.

3. Close your eye and place the mascara wand on top of the lashes at the base. Pull the wand through to remove any clumps.

Declumping Your Mascara

Are you trying to declump your mascara? Do not pump the wand into the mascara. This incorporates air into the product and dries it out. Instead, swirl the wand in the tube. If the mascara begins to get clumpy and swirling doesn't help, add a few eye drops to it. This will refresh the mascara.

OTHER EYELASH TOOLS AND TECHNIQUES

A couple coats of mascara isn't the only thing that can improve the look of your lashes.

The following tools and techniques help you achieve beautiful eyelashes beyond the mascara tube.

EYELASH CURLER

An eyelash curler is a tool used to curl your upper eyelashes prior to applying mascara or false eyelashes. It's normally made out of metal and has rubber strips on the curlers where the lashes are gripped. While using it is a fairly simple process, the following step-by-step shows you how to get the best results from your eyelash curler.

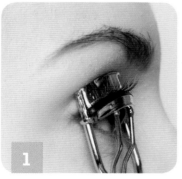

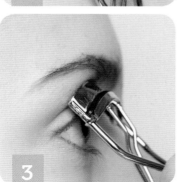

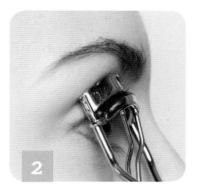

1. Place the eyelash curler close to your lash line.

2. Press the eyelash curler open and closed as you move the eyelash curler away from your eye.

3. Finish by pumping the eyelash curler upward. This encourages the lashes to curl away from your eyeball, giving your eyes a lift.

Longer-Lasting Curled Lashes

If you're looking for longer-lasting curled lashes, try heating your eyelash curler with a blow dryer for five seconds before use! The heat will curl your lashes just like a curling iron curls hair. However, be sure to not overheat the tool, or you'll risk burning your lashes or delicate eyelids.

EYELASH GLUE

Eyelash glue is a cosmetic adhesive that comes in white or black colors and is used to apply false eyelashes. In most cases, the glue dries clear after application. This glue is safe to use near your eyes and peels off quite easily.

FALSE EYELASHES

A must-have makeup staple between 1920 and 1960, false eyelashes were a must in every woman's makeup arsenal. However, that trend came to a halt during the relaxed 1970s era, when the natural look became popular. Today, false eyelashes are still a great choice when you want to glam up your look.

There are two types of lashes: strip and individual lashes. Made with human hair or synthetic materials, they come in many styles, colors, and lengths and are applied with eyelash glue. While they are not designed to be worn when showering, sleeping, or swimming, they can be used to add some drama, day or night.

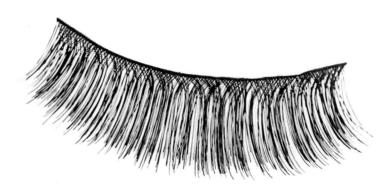

STRIP EYELASHES

Strip lashes come on a strip or band in different lengths and colors. If cared for properly, strip lashes can also be reused.

The following step-by-step guide assures a quick and clean application. While I use a bobby pin to press the lashes down, feel free to use tweezers or the end of your makeup brush. When you're ready to remove them, gently pull them off; you can use a gentle makeup cleanser to remove any excess glue.

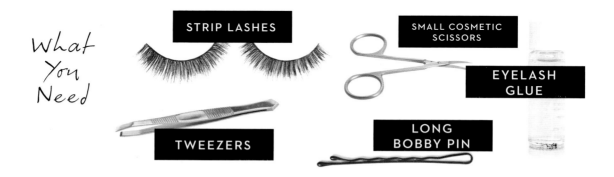

What You Need

STRIP LASHES

SMALL COSMETIC SCISSORS

EYELASH GLUE

TWEEZERS

LONG BOBBY PIN

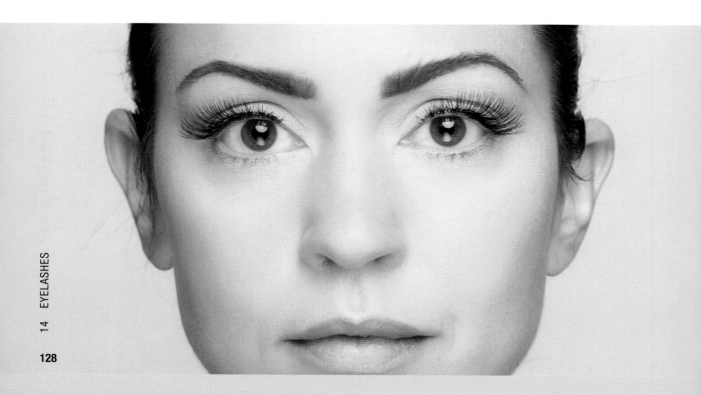

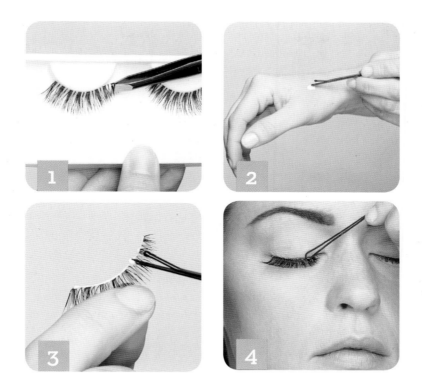

1. With a pair of tweezers, remove a false eyelash strip from its container. If the strip is too long, trim from the outside (wider) part of the lash strip.

2. Put a drop of eyelash glue on one end of the bobby pin.

3. Apply a thin line of glue on the eyelash with the bobby pin, and let the glue air-dry for about 30 seconds. If the glue is too wet, the strip will slide around.

4. Lay the strip as close to the lash line as possible. Press the strip lash down with the clean side of the bobby pin. Continue pressing the lash down in the center and work left to right until the lash has adhered.

OTHER EYELASH TOOLS AND TECHNIQUES

Eyelash Extensions

If you desire permanent full and long lashes, you might consider looking into eyelash extensions. They consist of sections of at least three false eyelashes glued together. Unlike false eyelashes, eyelash extensions aren't damaged by water from showering or swimming, making them a great option if you enjoy an active lifestyle. This lash type also gives you much more control in terms of how thick you want your lashes and where you put them.

Eyelash extensions come in three types: synthetic, mink, and silk. Whatever type you choose, they have to be applied by a professional. Extension lashes are permanent, not reusable, and can last up to six to eight weeks. Because extension eyelashes will fall out when you lose your natural lashes, it is recommended you get a touch-up every three to four weeks.

INDIVIDUAL EYELASHES

Unlike strip lashes, individual eyelashes typically come as one single lash or in a group of three lashes. They are used to fill in lashes where needed and can create a more natural look than strip lashes. The following takes you through how to apply them.

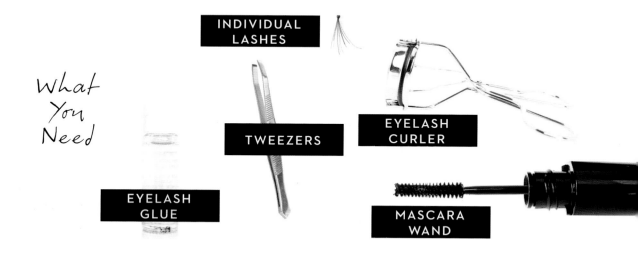

What You Need

INDIVIDUAL LASHES

TWEEZERS

EYELASH CURLER

EYELASH GLUE

MASCARA WAND

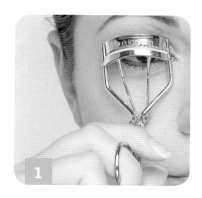 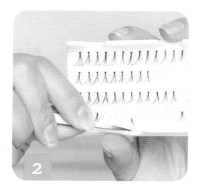 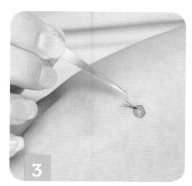

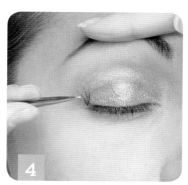 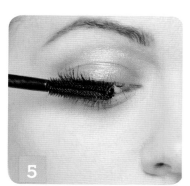

1. Curl your natural lashes to give them some bend. This makes them "hide" better with the fake lashes. Also, prep your lashes with one precoat of mascara. This also helps the lashes blend more seamlessly with the false lashes.

2. Using a clean set of tweezers or your fingers, grab one lash from your set of individual lashes.

3. Lightly dip the end of the lash into a dot of eyelash glue.

4. Starting from the outside of your eye, apply the lash right into your lash line using the tweezers. Let dry for a few seconds if you landed in the right spot, or take your time in moving it so the eyelash lines up with the rest of your natural lashes. Continue to fill in as many lashes as you need.

5. After you have applied the lashes and allowed the glue set and dry for a few minutes, gently comb through your lashes with a mascara wand. This ensures all the false and natural lashes aren't poking out in different directions.

OTHER EYELASH TOOLS AND TECHNIQUES

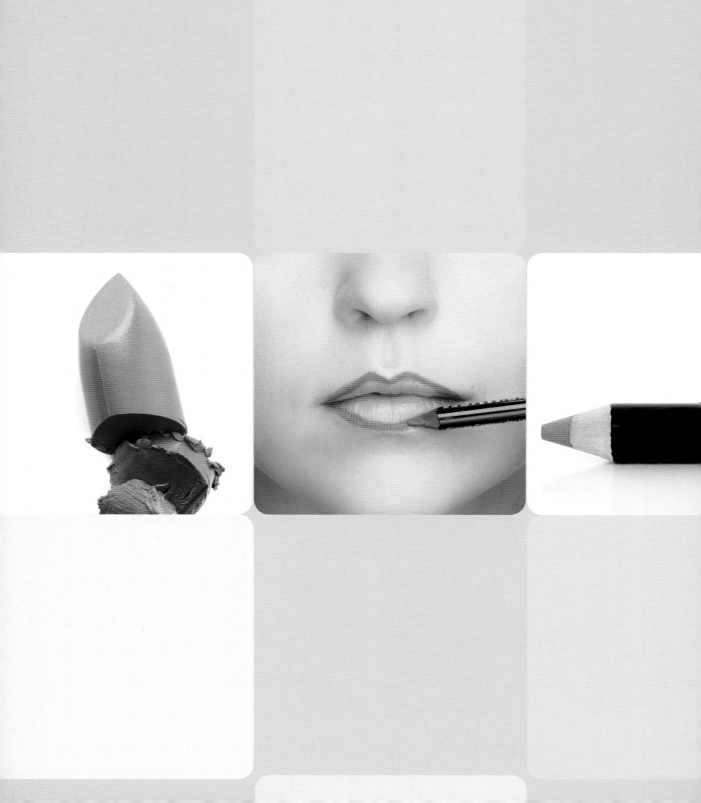

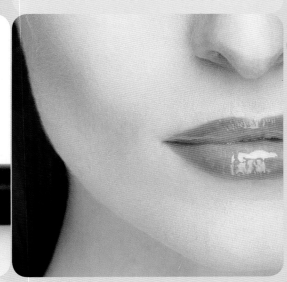

CHAPTER 15
LIPS

The lips are the second most important feature next to the eyes. Throughout the decades, there have been full red, hot pink, nude glossy, and soft dusty rose lip trends. Today, the market has dozens of different shades of lip colors. Taking the time to master the techniques to a great lip application allows you to complete a flawless look.

In this chapter, I discuss lip color products and how to choose the right lip color. I also talk about applying lip liner and correcting your lip shape to balance your face.

LIP COLOR PRODUCTS

Lip color products come in pencils, lipsticks, lip stains, and lip glosses.

Each type has its uses and advantages. Take a look at each type and see what you need for or would like to add to your makeup arsenal.

Lip pencil: This comes in a variety of shades and, like any cosmetic pencil, must be sharpened with a cosmetic pencil sharpener to keep its fine point. A lip pencil is not only great for outline work, but also for filling the lips to act as a base color.

Lipstick: This is the most common lip color application. It has a creamy consistency, is made from various forms of wax, and can contain emollients and oils for soft, healthy lips. Lipstick in tube form allows you to apply your lip color without any additional tools. However, cream lipstick, which comes in a pot or palette, requires a lip brush for application.

Fixing Broken Lipstick

Oops! Did you break your lipstick? Not to worry! Take a lighter or match (being careful not to burn yourself) and melt one end of the stick. Next, reattach the stick and hold it in place until dry. Your lipstick should be as good as new!

The Secret to Long-Lasting Lip Color

Looking for lip color with staying power? Using a lip pencil as a base color, line your lips and fill them in with the lip pencil. Next, apply a layer of lipstick and set with a matching powder eye shadow.

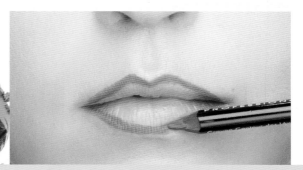

Lip stain: Made from a water and gel formula, it has a high pigment content and can last up to 18 hours. Lip stain is more difficult to remove than lipstick or lip pencil, requiring you to use a makeup remover or dish soap for best results.

Lip gloss: This comes in a gel consistency and is great for hydrating lips. Gloss comes in many complementary shades to lipstick, making it ideal to apply on top of matte lipstick for a juicy finish. Dabbing clear or tinted gloss in the center of the lip can also help create the illusion of fullness.

Lip balm: Created to help reduce cracked and chapped lips and to add moisture, lip balm is made with wax or paraffin and can contain flavors, pigments, and even sunscreen. Applying lip balm before applying lipstick will help your lipstick go on more smoothly.

Setting Your Lipstick

To set your lipstick, take a single-ply tissue and lay it across your finished lips. Apply setting powder to a brush, and then swipe the setting powder over the tissue. The powder will set your lips through the tissue.

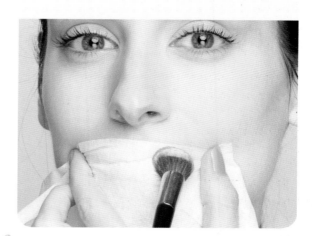

Getting the Last of Your Gloss

Many have dealt with the headache of being at the end of their lip gloss tube and unable to get the rest of the product out. However, you don't have to give it up to the trash. Dipping the tube into hot water will loosen up the product so you can access it.

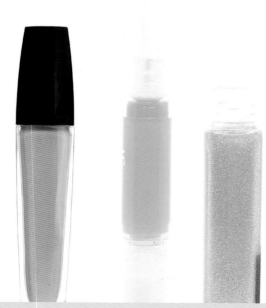

LIP COLOR PRODUCTS

Creating Your Own Lipstick Palette

With the following tools, you can actually create your own lipstick palette from lipsticks you have in separate containers.

Two different lipstick tubes

Large metal spoon

Candle

Empty and clean contact case

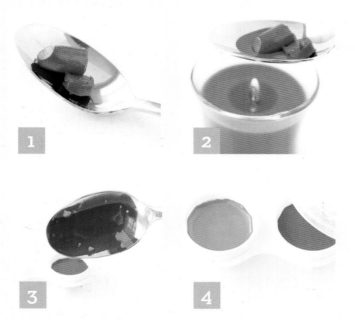

1. Place one color of lipstick in the large metal spoon.

2. Hold the metal spoon over the candle.

3. Once the lipstick becomes a liquid, pour it into one side of the contact case.

4. Repeat steps 1 through 3 with the second lipstick.

Voilà! You have created your own traveling lip palette. Apply with a lip brush and enjoy!

CHOOSING THE RIGHT LIP COLOR

Beauty product shelves are filled with many shades of lip colors.

How do you choose the right shade? One rule of thumb is to choose a lip color that is complementary to your cheek color; after all, you don't want your lip and cheek colors to be jarring.

Another consideration is your skin tone. You want a shade that doesn't wash you out or age you. The following are the best colors for different skin tones.

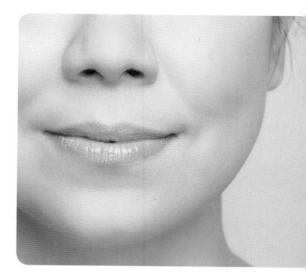

SKIN TONE	LIP COLOR	
FAIR	LIGHT PINK	LIGHT PEACH
	BEIGE	GOLDEN BROWN
MEDIUM	MEDIUM PINK	RED
	ORANGEY PEACH	APRICOT
OLIVE	DARK ROSE	DARK RED
	BERRY	DARK APRICOT
DARK	BROWNISH RED	DARK FUCHSIA
	DARK BERRY	GOLDEN BEIGE

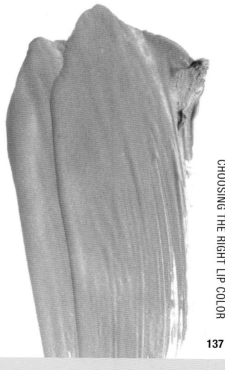

APPLYING LIP LINER

Are you having trouble lining your lips?

Do you simply need a process that's fast and easy? Follow these steps to get beautifully lined lips in no time!

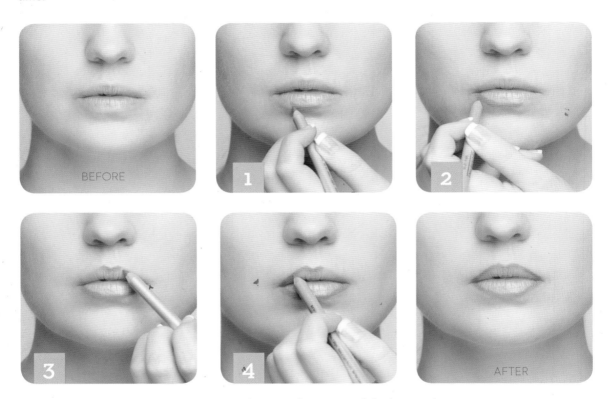

1. With your lip pencil, create a U shape at the center of the bottom lip.

2. Starting at one outside corner of the bottom lip, follow the lip line down to meet the center line. Repeat from the other outside corner.

3. On the upper lip, create a V shape within the cupid's bow.

4. Position your lip pencil at the corner of the mouth and travel up the lip, curving over and into the V. Repeat on the opposite side.

CREATING BALANCE BASED ON YOUR LIP SHAPE

Lips come in all shapes and sizes, but they basically boil down to these four types: average, wide, thin, and combination.

Your goal in your makeup application is to ensure your lips are in proportion to your face. Sometimes, to ensure your lips are proportional, you may need to correct your lip shape. The following shows you how to do this with foundation, lip pencil (sharpened, of course), and lip color or lip gloss.

AVERAGE

With average lips, the top and bottom lips are equal in size. In addition, the outer edges of the mouth align with the pupils of the eyes. Because the mouth is in proportion to the face, the lips need no correction. Therefore, simply apply your lip pencil and/or color by following the natural lip.

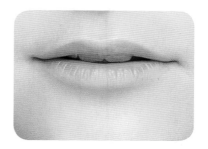

WIDE

With wide lips, the top and bottom lips are full and therefore too big for the face shape. The goal is to reduce the fullness of the lips, helping to balance them with the rest of the face. To correct the wide lip shape, follow these steps:

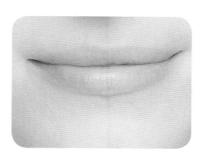

1. Cover the entire lip with your foundation color.

2. Using a lip pencil, draw a line just inside the lip line on the top and bottom lips.

3. Using the same lip pencil, fill inside the new lip line. Do not use a darker color, as it will only make the lips look fuller.

4. Apply lip color or gloss to finish the correction.

THIN

With thin lips, the top and bottom lips are thin and therefore too small for the face shape. The goal is to increase the fullness of the lips to restore balance. To correct the thin lip shape, follow these steps:

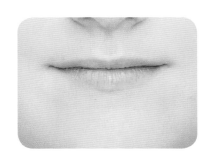

1. Cover the lip area with your foundation color.

2. With your lip pencil, draw a line just above the lip line on top and bottom.

3. Fill inside of the new lip line. You can choose to use a darker lip pencil color to create additional fullness.

4. Apply the lip color of your choice and a gloss at the center of the lip. The gloss placement gives a 3D effect to the lip.

COMBINATION

If you have a thin top lip and a full bottom lip (or vice versa), you have a combination lip. The goal is to address the different shapes so they are not only balanced in relation to your face, but also to each other. Follow the steps for correcting thin and wide lips based on the individual lip to achieve that look.

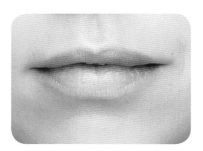

Avoiding Lip Stains on Your Glass

Would you like to keep your lipstick on your lips and not on the glass of wine you're enjoying? Here's an easy tip: Lick the rim of the glass before drinking. Miraculously, your lipstick stays where it should—on your lips!

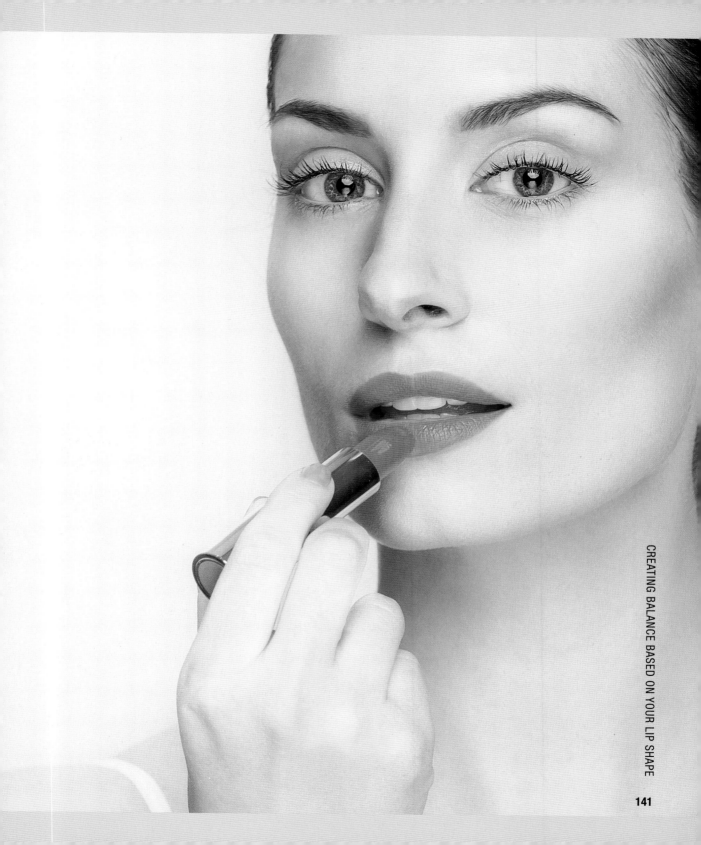

PART 3
BRINGING YOUR LOOK TOGETHER

CHAPTER 16
MAKEUP CHECKLIST

Before you get into trying some of the sample full-makeup applications of 10 classic looks, it's time to think about how to document your makeup looks. After all, you not only want to create a look that's best for you, but also remember it! That's where the makeup checklist comes in.

In this chapter, I take you through the two important components of the makeup checklist: the profile sheet and the face sheet.

PROFILE SHEET

I created this profile sheet as a tool for you to better understand your unique face and how your face relates to your makeup choices.

For example, you will often find it difficult to replicate a makeup look you watch online or read in a magazine. That is because the design was on the model in the tutorial, who had her own unique face profile. A good makeup artist has the ability to adapt techniques with each face they encounter. Having a clear understanding of your own face fingerprint will make replicating these looks that much easier.

The first part of the profile sheet has you identify your unique facial features so you can know what type of highlighting and contouring you'll need to do to create the most appealing look. In the case of copying a model's look, if you have deep-set eyes and the model doesn't, you have to consider how you apply the same eye shadows in a personally flattering way.

The second half of the profile sheet evaluates your skin type and the basic makeup choices that coordinate with your skin type. This will become your guide for everyday makeup foundation. Keep in mind, skin concerns and color can change based on the time of year—you may have lighter, dryer skin in the winter and darker, breakout-prone skin in the summer. Therefore, a few items on this profile sheet may change throughout the year.

If necessary, go back through the book as you fill out the profile sheet to ensure you're making the most accurate choices.

Additional Copies

Want additional copies of this sheet? Go to idiotsguides.com/everydaymakeupsecrets to print off as many as you need.

NAME:_____   AGE:_____

1.	**FACE SHAPE**	Oval	Oblong (Rectangle)	Heart	Diamond	Round	Square

2.	**EYE SHAPE**	Almond	Wide Set	Close Set	Deep Set	Prominent	Small
		Monolid	Hooded	Upturned	Downturned		

3.	**EYE COLOR**	Blue	Green	Brown	Hazel

4.	**EYEBROWS**	Round	Angled	Soft Angled	Curved	Flat

5.	**NOSE**	Natural	Wide	Thin	Long	Short

6.	**LIPS**	Average	Wide	Thin	Combination

7.	**SKIN TYPE**	Normal	Oily	Dry	Combination	Sensitive

8.	**AREAS OF CONCERN**	Acne	Rosacea	Dark Circles	Dark Spots/ Age Spots	Scars	Redness

9.	**SKIN TONE**	Warm	Cool

10.	**PRIMER**	Clear	Red	Green	Yellow	Purple

11.	**FOUNDATION**	Cream	Liquid	Tinted	Pressed Powder	Mineral

FACE SHEET

Now that you have a better understanding of what works for your face and skin type, you can begin building your makeup design.

A handy tool to have as part of your makeup checklist is a face sheet, something you may have seen a makeup artist use at the makeup counter at some point. Basically, you include the following information on a face sheet:

- **Foundation/concealer:** Includes primers, concealers, foundations, or setting powders

- **Corrective makeup:** Includes highlights and contours

- **Eyes:** Includes eye shadows, eyeliners, mascara, or false eyelashes

- **Cheeks:** Includes cheek colors

- **Lips:** Includes lip pencil, lipstick, or lip gloss

To fill out this sheet, use your finger, a brush, or a disposable applicator to apply makeup on the sheet based on what you use to create your look. You can then label the product used in the free space provided. I would suggest applying makeup on the face sheet exactly how you applied it to your face so you more accurately see how the colors looked.

The next page shows you a blank face sheet. If you'd like to see one filled out, check out any of the looks in Chapter 17.

Additional Copies

If you would like additional copies of this sheet, go to idiotsguides.com/everydaymakeupsecrets to print off as many as you need.

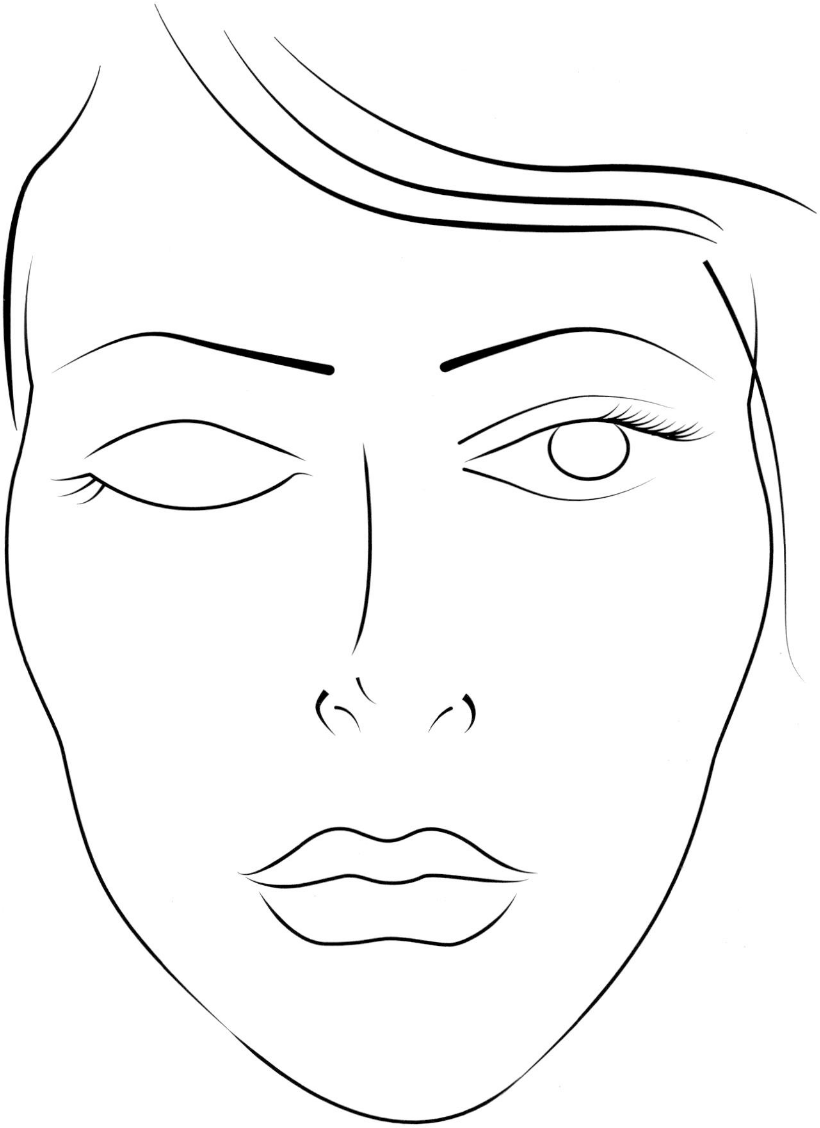

FOUNDATION/CONCEALER

_____

_____

_____

CORRECTIVE MAKEUP

_____

_____

EYES

_____

_____

_____

_____

_____

CHEEKS

_____

_____

LIPS

_____

_____

FACE SHEET

149

CHAPTER 17
TEN CLASSIC LOOKS

Now that you have the knowledge, the tools, and the secrets, let's put a look together! In this chapter, I provide 10 makeup applications I feel stand the test of time: daytime natural, elegant evening, dramatic evening, 1940s bridal, 1950s chic, 1970s bronze, metallic smoky eye, all about the lips, mature mineral, and youthful glitter.

Each look includes a completed face sheet and profile sheet for each model, in order to help guide you in mapping out the look for your unique face shape, facial features, and skin type. As you'll see, even a little makeup can make a big impact!

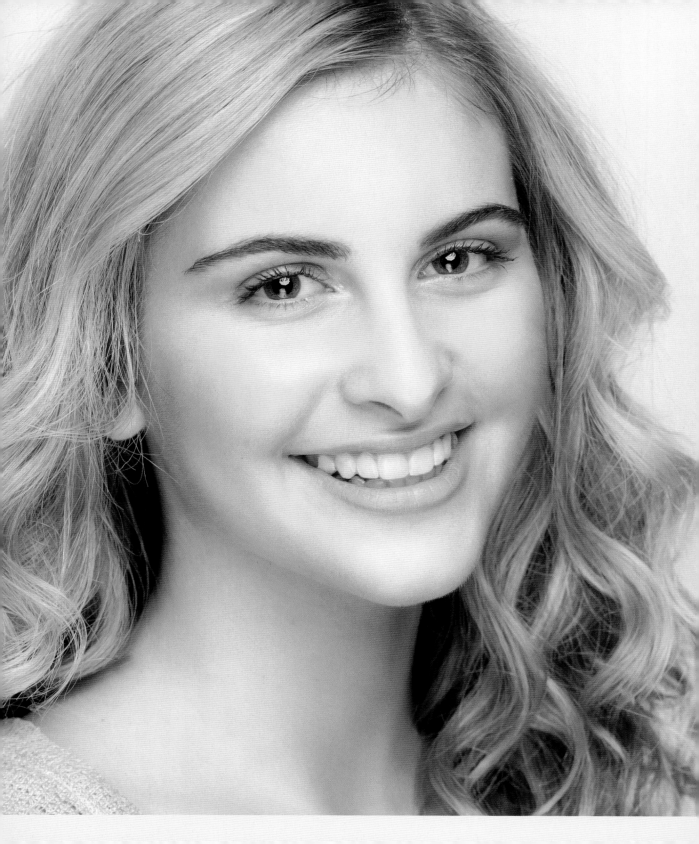

DAYTIME
natural

Makeup doesn't have to be complicated. The key to a daytime look is keeping your makeup light and translucent. A simple eye, a little mascara, and a glossy lip are all you need for a beautifully natural look.

DAYTIME NATURAL
FACE SHEET

FOUNDATION/CONCEALER:
Concealer (half-shade lighter)
Tinted liquid foundation

CORRECTIVE MAKEUP:
Cream highlight

EYES:
Ivory eye shadow
Taupe eye shadow
Dark brown mascara

CHEEKS:
Peach-pink blush

LIPS:
Peach-pink jumbo cream
lip pencil
Clear lip gloss

DAYTIME NATURAL
PROFILE SHEET

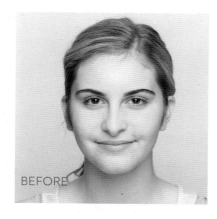

BEFORE

NAME: *Josie*

AGE: *16*

FACE SHAPE: *oval*

EYE SHAPE: *deep set*

EYE COLOR: *green*

EYEBROWS: *curved*

NOSE: *natural*

LIPS: *average*

SKIN TYPE: *dry*

AREAS OF
CONCERN: *none*

SKIN TONE: *warm*

PRIMER: *none*

FOUNDATION: *liquid*

Tools

Disposable latex sponge

Blush brush

Large eye shadow brush

Medium eye shadow brush

Eyelash curler

Disposable mascara wand

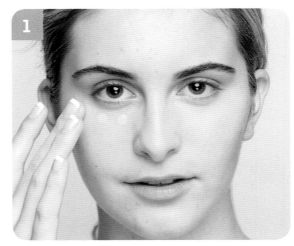

1 Apply concealer that's a half-shade lighter under the eyes and around the nose and lips to conceal any redness or trouble spots.

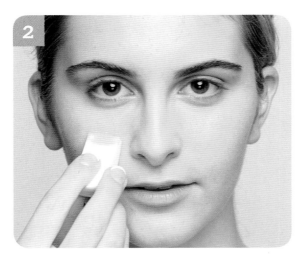

2 Using a sponge, apply tinted liquid foundation. The tinted moisturizer helps create a sheer, natural look.

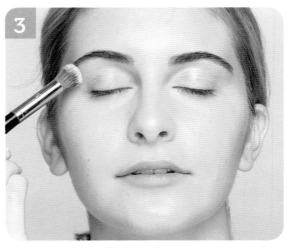

3 Apply ivory eye shadow all over each eyelid, starting at the brow bone and working your way down to the upper lashline.

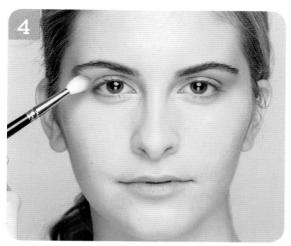

4

Apply a matte medium taupe eye shadow in each crease.

Eye Shadow for Deep-Set Eyes

Josie has deep-set eyes, so using eye shadow highlight helps bring her eyes forward. If you have deep-set eyes, you can do the same and use the same shadow under the eye and into the upper cheek to add a highlight. Avoid using dark colors on the eyelids, as that will make your eyes appear they're set back even deeper.

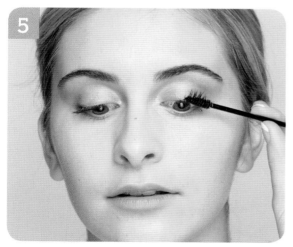

5

After prepping the eyelashes with an eyelash curler, apply dark brown mascara on the top lashes only.

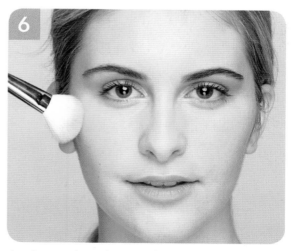

6

Apply peach-pink cream blush to the cheeks, making sure to follow the natural cheekbones. Dust a cream highlight on the cheeks for a bright, dewy look.

DAYTIME NATURAL

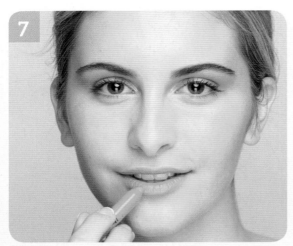

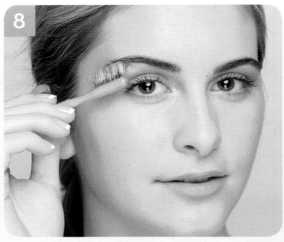

Fill the lips with a peach-pink jumbo cream lip pencil to enhance the natural lip color. You can add a bit of shine to the lips with a clear lip gloss.

Refresh the eyebrows by brushing them with a disposable mascara wand or other brush tool.

Creating a Dewy Look

If you want a natural "dewy" look, choose a liquid foundation, cream highlighter, and cream cheek color. Cream makeup will look more supple and moisturized than powder. The exception, of course, is if you have oily skin; avoid creams, since they'll be more likely to break out your skin.

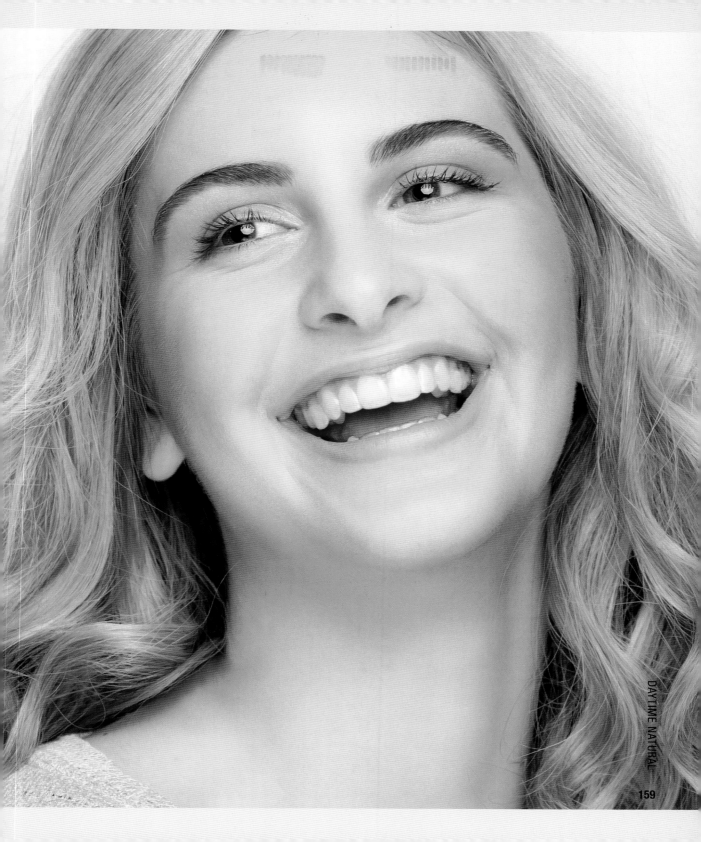

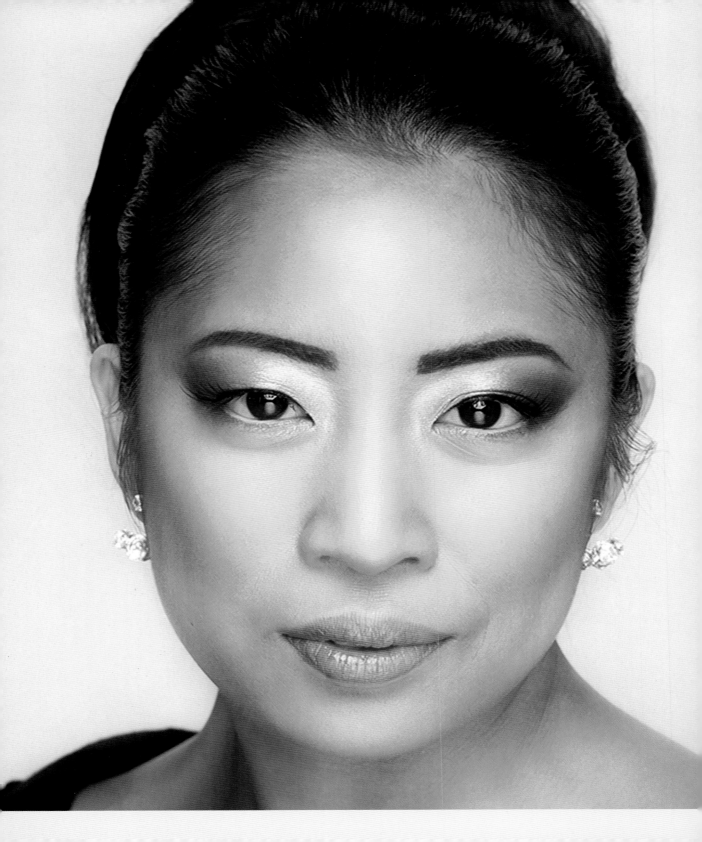

ELEGANT
evening

This full makeup application with a focus on the eye is perfect for special occasions, such as an evening wedding, holiday party, or gala event. Because the lighting at a formal evening event tends to be subdued, using a shimmer eye shadow can reflect the lighting in a way that gives you a romantic glow. You can even add some strip eyelashes to ramp up this elegant look.

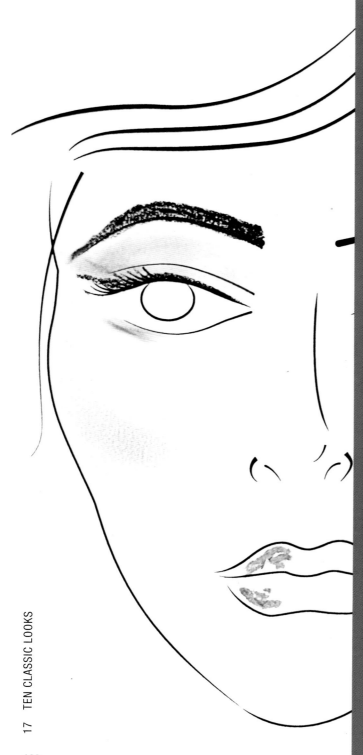

ELEGANT EVENING
FACE SHEET

FOUNDATION/CONCEALER:
Concealer (half-shade lighter)
Full-coverage liquid foundation

CORRECTIVE MAKEUP:
Cream highlight
Brown cream eye shadow
Tinted setting powder

EYES:
Black eyebrow pencil
Eye shadow (one shade lighter)
Shimmer taupe eye shadow
Pale yellow shimmer eye shadow
Dark brown matte eye shadow
Flesh-colored eye pencil
Black liquid eyeliner
Black mascara

CHEEKS:
Dusty rose blush

LIPS:
Matte raspberry jumbo lip pencil
Nude lip gloss

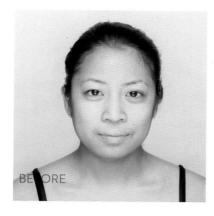

BEFORE

ELEGANT EVENING
PROFILE SHEET

NAME: Arianne

AGE: 23

FACE SHAPE: round

EYE SHAPE: monolid

EYE COLOR: brown

EYEBROWS: soft angled

NOSE: wide

LIPS: wide

SKIN TYPE: dry and sensitive

AREAS OF CONCERN: none

SKIN TONE: warm

PRIMER: none

FOUNDATION: liquid

Tools

Powder brush

Blush brush

Large eye shadow brush

Medium eye shadow brush

Eyelash curler

False strip eyelashes and cosmetic scissors
(optional)

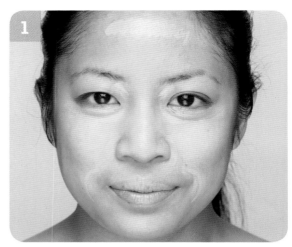

Apply concealer that's a half-shade lighter under the eyes, around the nose, on the "parentheses" around the lips, on the forehead, and on the chin.

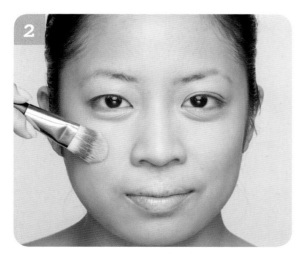

Apply full-coverage liquid foundation.

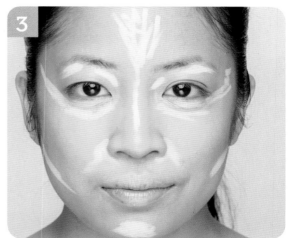

Apply cream highlight under the cheeks, along the nose and middle of the forehead, around the nose, under the eyes and eyebrows, and on the chin.

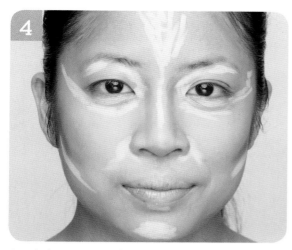

Apply brown eye shadow contour along the cheekbones, sides of the nose, tip of the nose, and jawline and above the hairline along the temple.

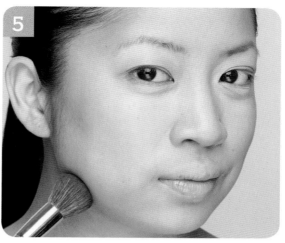

Blend the highlight and contour by brushing on tinted setting powder.

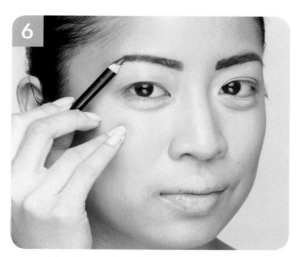

Use a black pencil to fill and shape your brows. This will create dynamic, soft-angled brows.

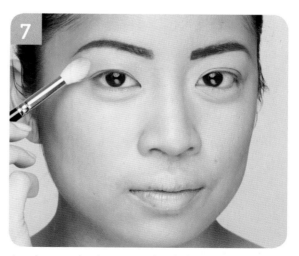

Apply eye shadow one shade lighter than your natural skin tone under the brow bones and down into the corner of the eyes.

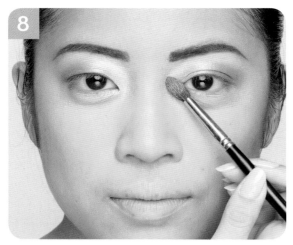

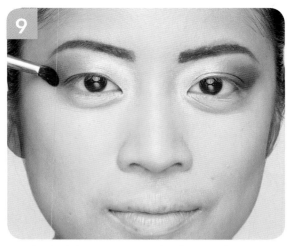

Apply shimmer taupe eye shadow from the tear ducts and over the eyelids. Open your eyes and reapply. Apply pale yellow shimmer eye shadow in the inside corner of the eye, stopping just before the center.

Apply dark brown matte shadow to the outside corner of the eyelids.

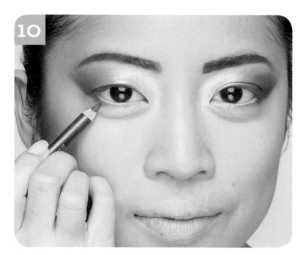

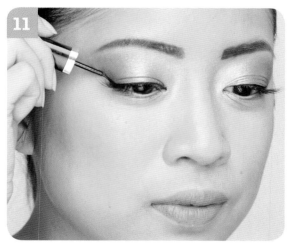

Apply a flesh-colored pencil followed by a brown pencil onto the water line to give the illusion of having wider eyes.

Apply a thin line of black liquid eyeliner starting in the corner of each eye, following the natural lash line around; end with a thin wing tip.

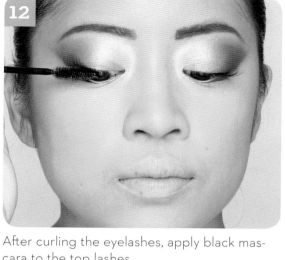

After curling the eyelashes, apply black mascara to the top lashes.

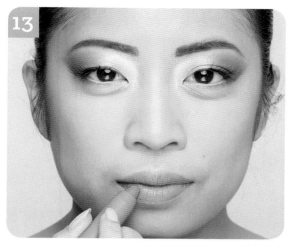

Apply dusty rose blush to the cheeks. Fill and line the lips with a matte raspberry jumbo lip pencil. Dab lip gloss (either nude or a similar color to the lip color) onto the center of the lips for highlight.

Optional Strip Lash

Before putting on mascara, add half of a false strip eyelash to the corner of the eyes to fill out your lashes. Simply cut a strip lash in half and use the fuller half on the upper lash line.

Making Your Eyes Appear Larger

To make your eyes appear larger, apply a white liner on the lower water line. Next, directly underneath the white line, apply a brown or black eyeliner. Doing so will give the illusion of a larger eye.

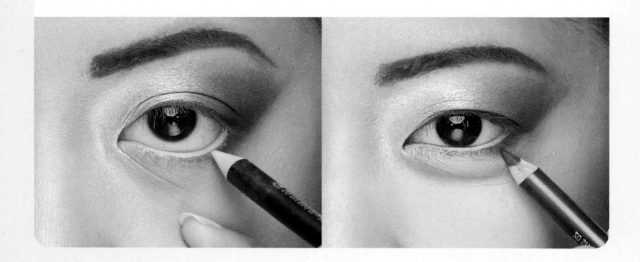

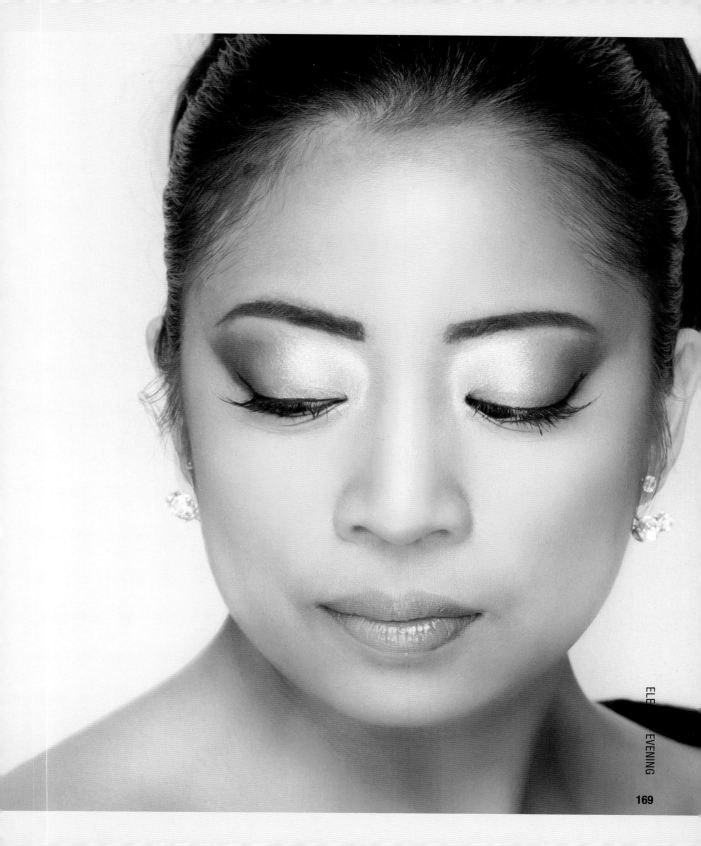

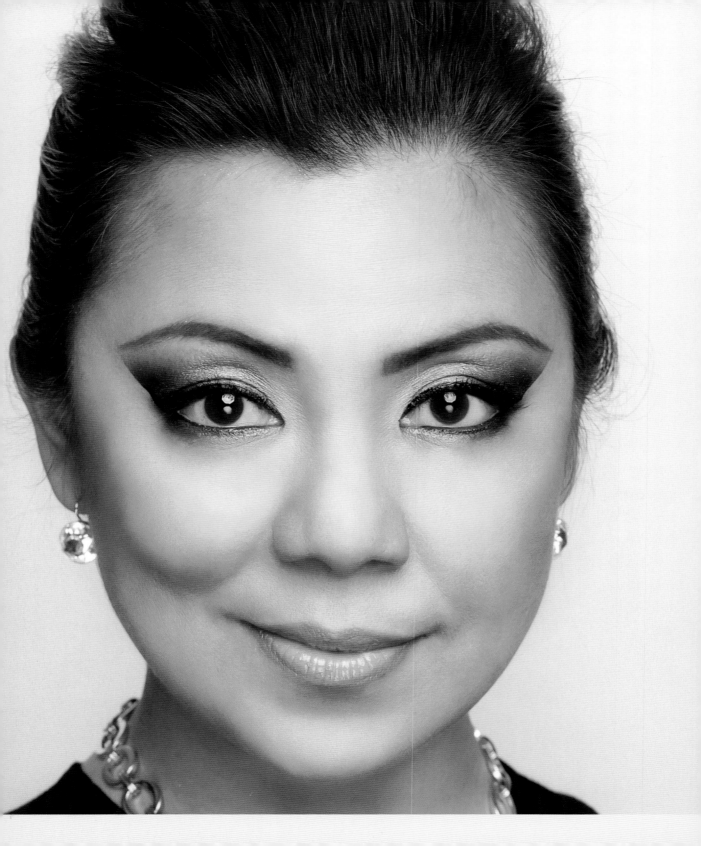

DRAMATIC
evening

When you are going out to a club, a bachelorette party, or anyplace you can let loose, you have a chance to really go bold with your makeup! Like the elegant evening makeup, the lighting in most nighttime venues is darker, making it a prime opportunity to create drama with your look. For this makeup, you'll make the eyes your showy statement piece.

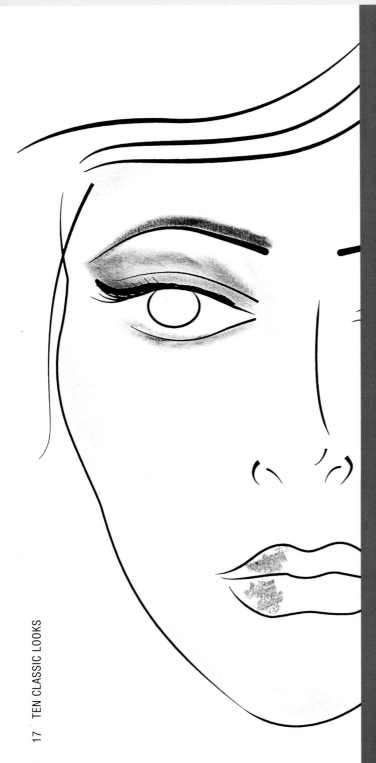

DRAMATIC EVENING
FACE SHEET

FOUNDATION/CONCEALER:
Concealer
Full-coverage cream foundation

CORRECTIVE MAKEUP:
Cream highlight pencil

EYES:
Dark brown eyebrow pencil
Pale gold shimmer eye shadow
Bronze shimmer eye shadow
Teal shimmer eye shadow
Midnight blue shimmer eye
shadow
Black liquid eyeliner
Black mascara

CHEEKS:
Dusty rose blush

LIPS:
Flesh-colored lip pencil
Flesh-colored lip gloss

DRAMATIC EVENING
PROFILE SHEET

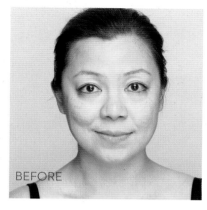

BEFORE

NAME:	Nathalie
AGE:	39
FACE SHAPE:	round
EYE SHAPE:	monolid
EYE COLOR:	brown
EYEBROWS:	soft angled
NOSE:	wide
LIPS:	wide
SKIN TYPE:	oily
AREAS OF CONCERN:	dark circles
SKIN TONE:	warm
PRIMER:	clear
FOUNDATION:	cream

Tools

Disposable latex sponge

Blush brush

Large eye shadow brush

Medium eye shadow brush

Scotch tape

Index card

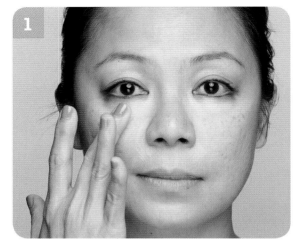

Apply concealer under the eyes, around the nose, and wherever else you have redness.

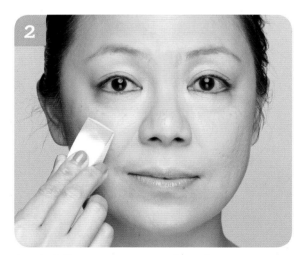

Apply full-coverage cream foundation.

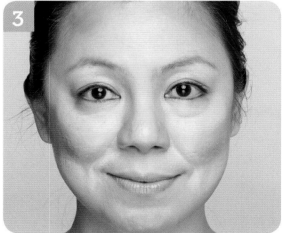

Apply highlight and contour to the cheeks, nose, jawline, and forehead. Blend highlight and contour into the foundation with a damp sponge.

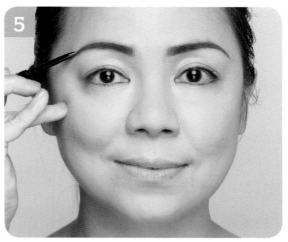

Brush a soft duty rose blush between highlight and contour, following the natural line of the cheeks.

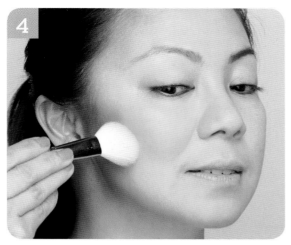

With a dark brown pencil, start filling in the eyebrows from the inside corner of the eye, creating "hair strokes" straight up and angled toward the natural brow shape. The brows should be slightly fuller near the nose and thinner through the arch and end of the brow.

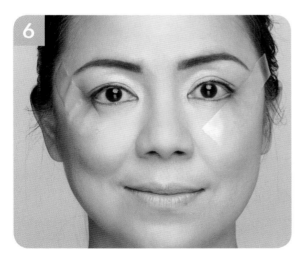

Place Scotch tape along the outside of the eyes, starting at the outside corner and angling to the end of the eyebrows; this will help you with placement. Apply pale gold shimmer eye shadow from the corner of each eye and follow up across the entire eyebrow, ending at the brow bone to create a crease.

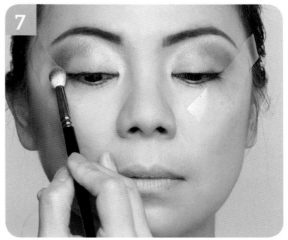

Apply a shimmer bronze eye shadow under the highlight (on the upper crease) for each eye.

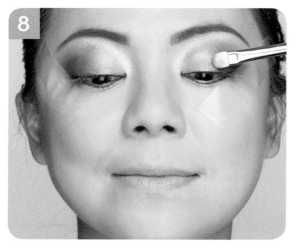

Apply teal shimmer eye shadow on the lash lines and into the crease of each eyelid.

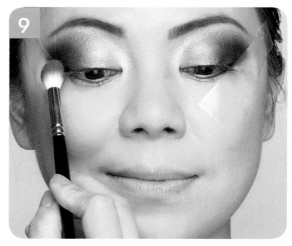

Apply midnight blue shimmer shadow on the end of the lash line, swooping up along the edge to create a smoky eye.

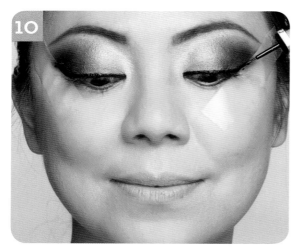

Line each eye with black liquid eyeliner by following the lash line and traveling up the side of the tape. Apply black eyeliner in the lower water lines for a dramatic look. When finished, gently remove the tape.

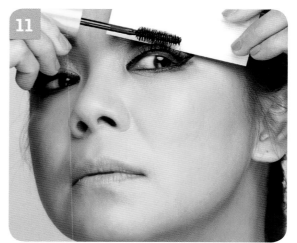

Load up the eyelashes with very black mascara. You can place an index card on the eyelids to avoid creating streaks on them.

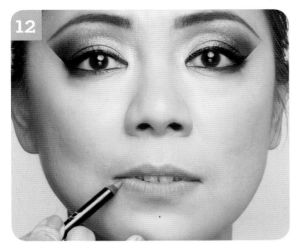

Use flesh-colored lip pencil to fill in the lips.

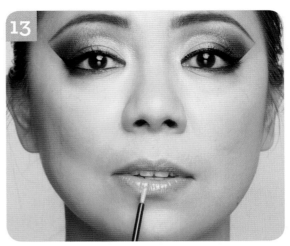

Apply flesh-colored lip gloss over the lip pencil.

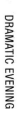

The Scotch Tape Method

Here's a tip for a flawless eye shadow application:

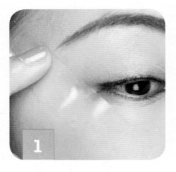

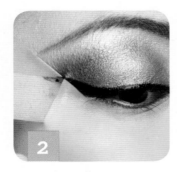

1 Place a piece of scotch tape at an angle from the outside corner of the eye to the end of the eyebrow and apply your eye shadows.

2 When you are finished, carefully remove the tape.

3 As you can see, you're left with a clean shadow line. People will think you've had your makeup done by a professional!

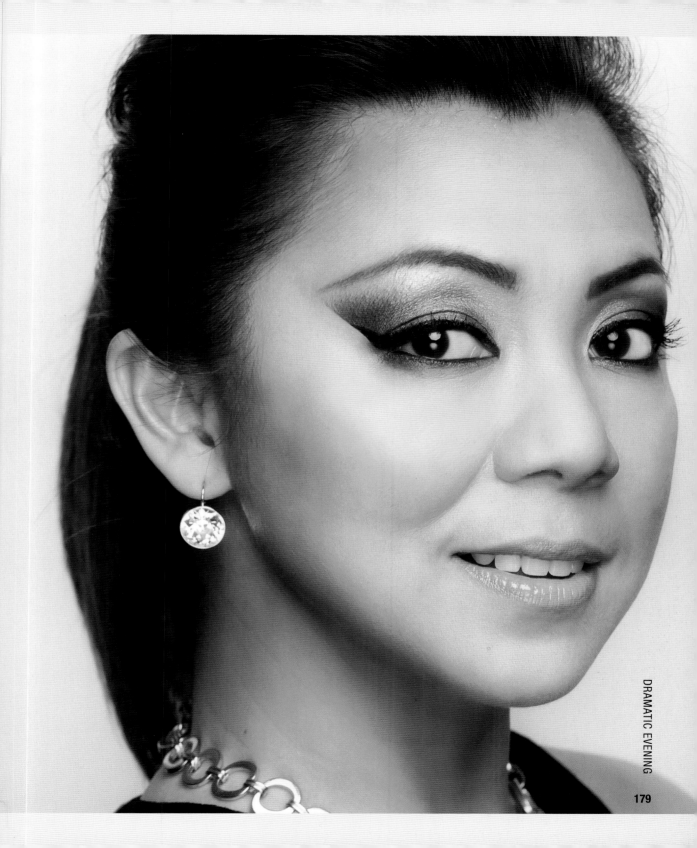

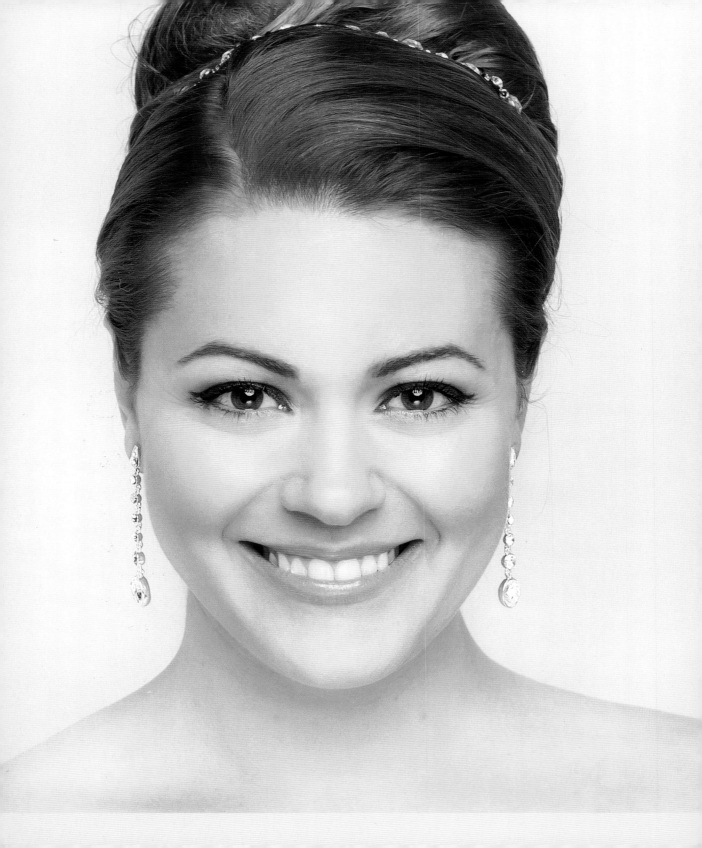

1940s
bridal

What woman doesn't want to look like a princess on the happiest day of her life? One of the greatest joys of a makeup artist is to transform a bride. The quintessential bride makeup is a 1940s look—emphasis on the eyes, great eyebrows, dusty rose cheeks, and luscious lips. Whether you're getting married or simply wanting a gorgeous but not dramatic look, this makeup is beautifully timeless.

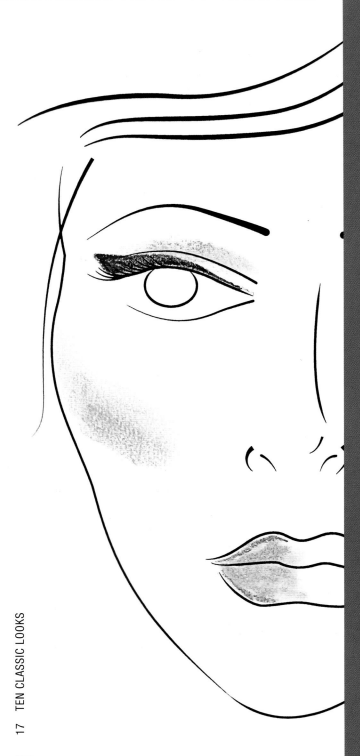

1940s BRIDAL
FACE SHEET

FOUNDATION/CONCEALER:
Concealer
Liquid foundation

CORRECTIVE MAKEUP:
Light brown contour
Ivory highlight

EYES:
Ivory eye shadow
Rose-gold shimmer eye
shadow
Black mascara
Dark brown gel pot eyeliner
Medium brown eyebrow pencil

CHEEKS:
Deep rose-pink blush

LIPS:
Nude lip pencil
Deep rose-pink lipstick

1940s BRIDAL
PROFILE SHEET

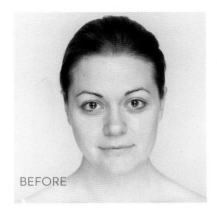

BEFORE

NAME: Betsy

AGE: 29

FACE SHAPE: oval

EYE SHAPE: average

EYE COLOR: light brown

EYEBROWS: soft angled

NOSE: natural

LIPS: wide

SKIN TYPE: dry

AREAS OF CONCERN: dark circles/redness

SKIN TONE: warm

PRIMER: none

FOUNDATION: liquid

Tools

Disposable latex sponge

Blush brush

Powder brush

Large eye shadow brush

Medium eye shadow brush

Angle brush

Reducing Redness

If concealer isn't helping the redness in Step 1, you can apply a thin amount of green primer to further reduce the redness.

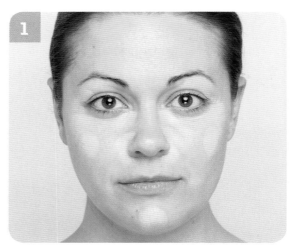

Apply concealer under the eye, around the nose, on the chin, and wherever else you need to reduce redness.

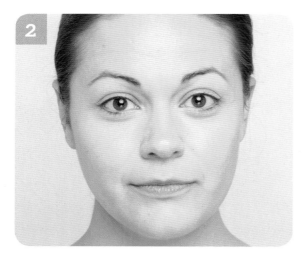

Apply matte liquid foundation all over the face.

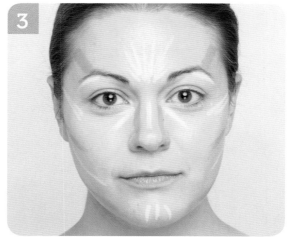

Apply light brown contour to the sides of the nose, under the cheekbone, and to the jawline and temple. Apply ivory highlight down the nose, ending before the tip of the nose. Add highlight on the forehead and chin, upper cheekbones, and hollows of the cheeks, and under the brow bones.

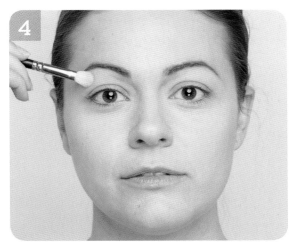

Use medium brown pencil to fill in the eyebrows. Apply matte ivory eye shadow under the brows and down to the tear ducts.

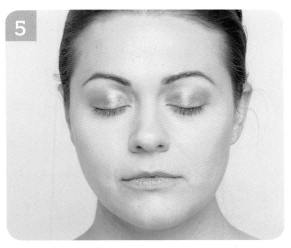

Apply rose-gold shimmer eye shadow on the entire eyelid, and then slightly into the crease, of each eye.

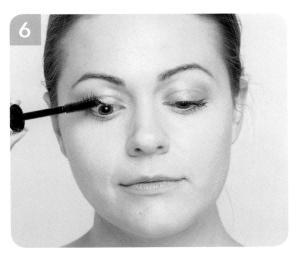

Apply black mascara to the top lashes.

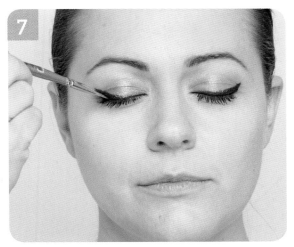

Apply dark brown gel pot eyeliner. Start with a thin line on each inner lash and move along the lash line, creating a thicker line as you move toward the end. Load up the eyelashes with very black mascara.

1940s BRIDAL

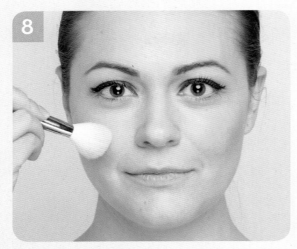

8

Apply deep rose-pink blush on the apples of the cheeks.

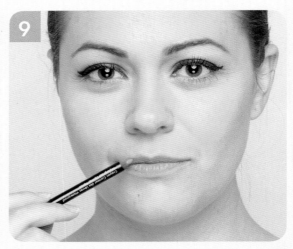

9

Lightly line and then fill in the lips with nude lip pencil.

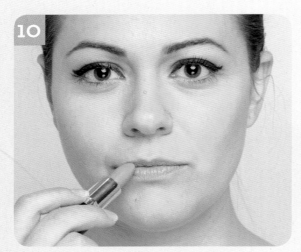

10

With your finger, lightly apply a deep rose-pink lipstick.

Applying Mascara

You can place a plastic spoon on the eyelids to avoid creating streaks on them.

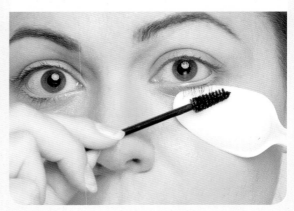

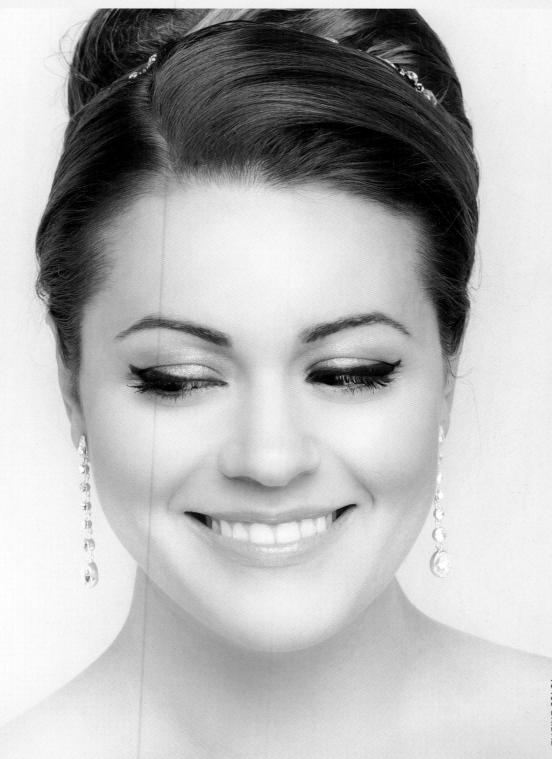

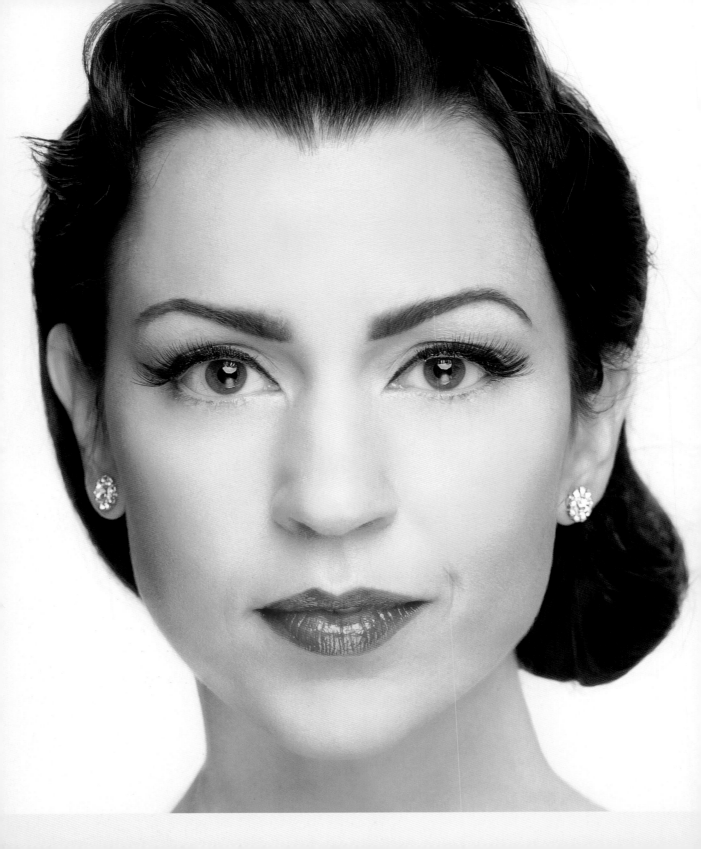

1950s
chic

Makeup looks are typically variations of trends from past decades. However, the 1950s has stood the test of time. Characteristics of the look continue to be black-lined eyes with a strong, winged tip and a bright red lip. If you want to fully emulate the 1950s look, your foundation should be matte and a half shade to full shade lighter than your natural skin tone.

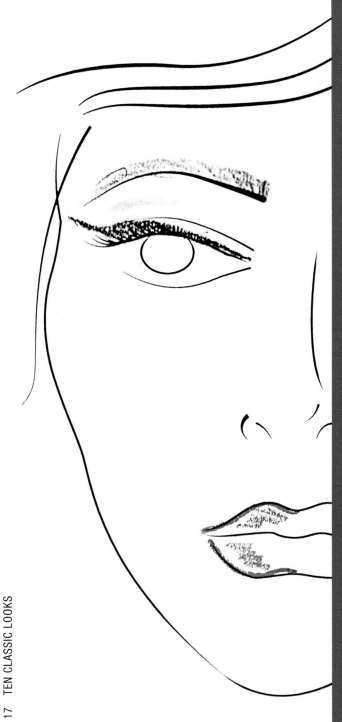

1950s CHIC
FACE SHEET

FOUNDATION/CONCEALER:
Cream concealer (one shade lighter)
Cream foundation

CORRECTIVE MAKEUP:
Taupe contour
Cream highlight
Tinted setting powder (fair)

EYES:
Vanilla matte eye shadow
Light taupe matte eye shadow
Dark brown eyebrow pencil
Black mascara
False strip eyelashes and eye-
lash glue (optional)
Black gel pot eyeliner

CHEEKS:
None

LIPS:
Red lip pencil
Bright red lipstick
Red lip gloss

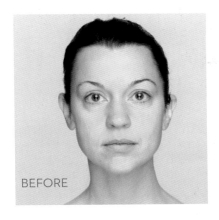

BEFORE

1950s CHIC
PROFILE SHEET

NAME: *Jill*

AGE: *36*

FACE SHAPE: *oblong (rectangle)*

EYE SHAPE: *almond*

EYE COLOR: *brown*

EYEBROWS: *soft angled*

NOSE: *natural*

LIPS: *average*

SKIN TYPE: *normal*

AREAS OF CONCERN: *dark circles*

SKIN TONE: *warm*

PRIMER: *none*

FOUNDATION: *cream*

Tools

Foundation brush

Disposable latex sponge

Powder brush

Large eye shadow brush

Medium eye shadow brush

Angle brush

Cotton swab with makeup remover
(optional)

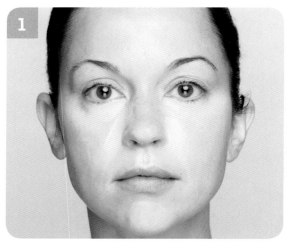

Apply cream concealer that's a full shade lighter than your natural skin tone under the eye, around the corners of the nose and lips, and wherever there is redness.

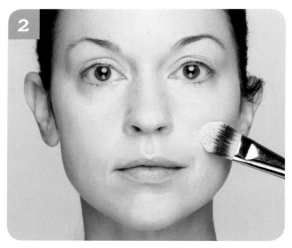

Apply full-coverage matte cream foundation all over the face.

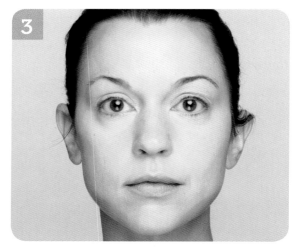

Using a taupe powder, contour the hollows of the cheekbones, the recession of the hairline, and just above the jawline to soften the edges.

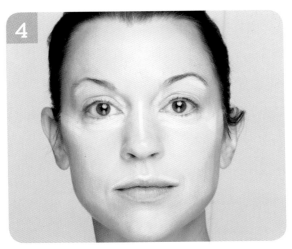

Apply cream highlight under the eyes; to the tops of the cheekbones; and to the lips, brow bones, and inside corners of the eyes.

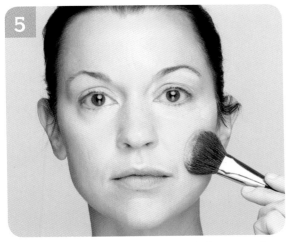

Blend highlight and contour with fair-tinted setting powder.

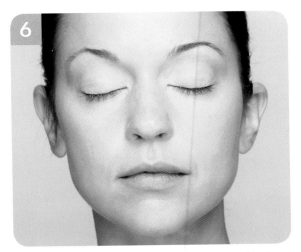

Apply vanilla eye shadow on the lid and light taupe eye shadow on the outside crease.

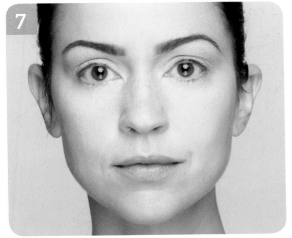

Take a dark brown eyebrow pencil and fill the brows from the inside corner of the eye around, creating "hair strokes" straight up and slightly angled toward the natural brow shape. For a full brow, fill slightly fuller near the nose and thinner through the arch and end of the brow.

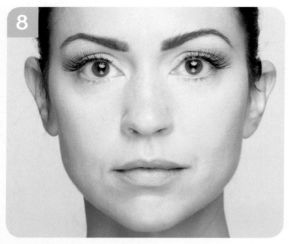

Apply multiple coats of black mascara.

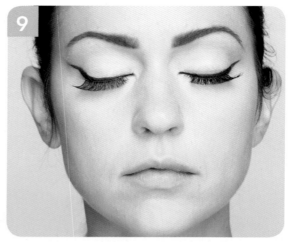

Apply a thin line of black gel pot eyeliner to each eye starting on the inside corner of the eye. Gradually make the line thicker as you line along the top, and end with a winged tip. If necessary, use a cotton swab with oil-free makeup remover to define the line.

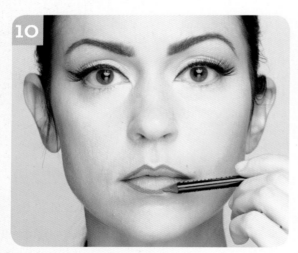

Apply red lip pencil, following the natural line of the lips.

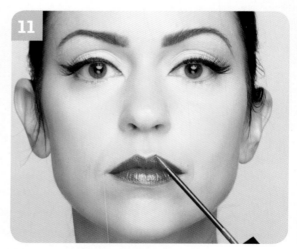

Apply bright red lipstick and finish with bright red lip gloss.

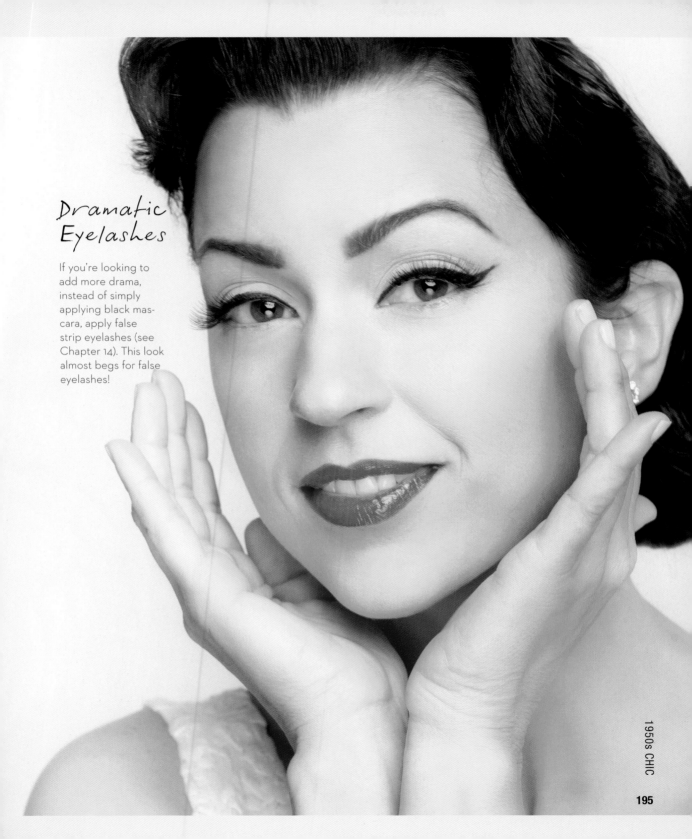

Dramatic Eyelashes

If you're looking to add more drama, instead of simply applying black mascara, apply false strip eyelashes (see Chapter 14). This look almost begs for false eyelashes!

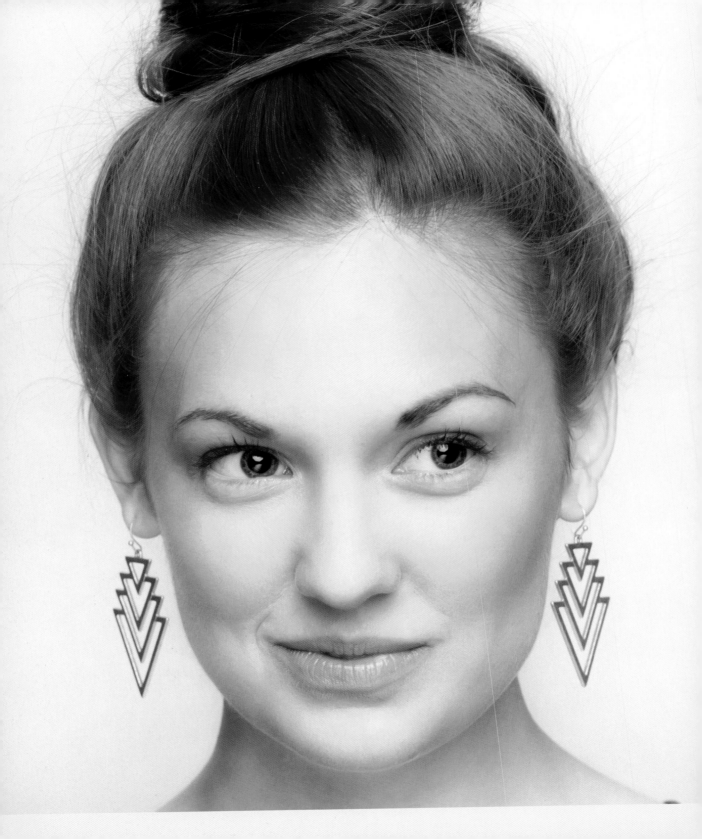

1970s
bronze

The 1970s introduced the natural, sun-kissed look. Thankfully, you don't have to sit in a tanning booth to get this look. You can simply use copper tones and a bronzer to achieve a similar look without the sun's damaging UV rays. In the end, you'll have skin that looks translucent and dewy. You can then finish off the look with a beautiful glossy lip.

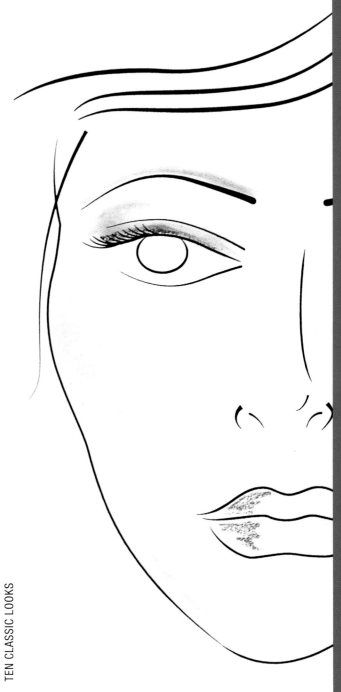

1970s BRONZE

FACE SHEET

FOUNDATION/CONCEALER:
Green cream primer
Sheer liquid foundation

CORRECTIVE MAKEUP:
None

EYES:
Medium brown eyebrow pencil
Medium copper cream eye shadow
Soft gold shimmer eye shadow
Brown eyeliner pencil
Brown mascara

CHEEKS:
Bronzer

LIPS:
Apricot lip pencil
Apricot lip gloss

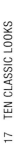

1970s BRONZE
PROFILE SHEET

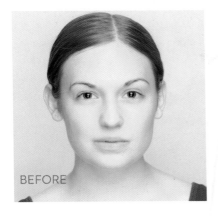

BEFORE

NAME:	Audrey
AGE:	25
FACE SHAPE:	square
EYE SHAPE:	downturned
EYE COLOR:	blue
EYEBROWS:	soft angled
NOSE:	natural
LIPS:	wide
SKIN TYPE:	combination
AREAS OF CONCERN:	redness
SKIN TONE:	warm
PRIMER:	green
FOUNDATION:	liquid

Tools

Medium eye shadow brush

Powder brush

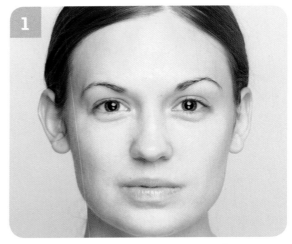

Apply green cream primer to neutralize any redness under the eyes.

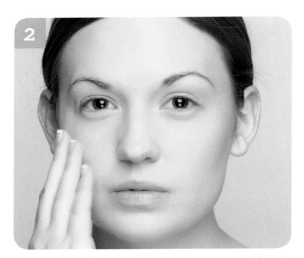

Apply sheer foundation, making sure to blend it into the primer.

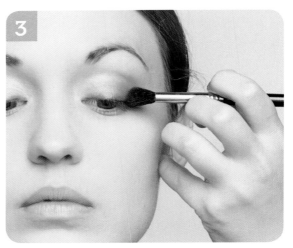

Apply medium copper eye shadow on the eyelids and soft gold shimmer eye shadow on the brow bones. Use a medium brown eyebrow pencil to fill in the brows.

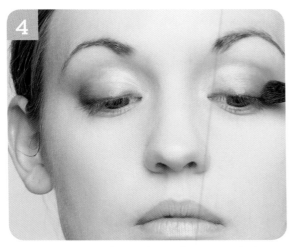

4

Apply brown eyeliner along the upper lash lines. Run the eye shadow brush across the eyeliner to soften the line, creating a more natural look.

Lining Downturned Eyes

Do you have downturned eyes like Audrey? Move the eyeliner up at the end to give the illusion of an upturned eye.

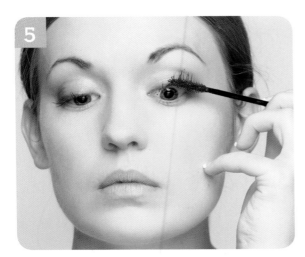

5

Finish the eyes by applying brown mascara on the top lashes.

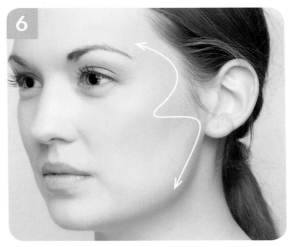

6

Apply bronzer starting at the temple and curving down into the cheekbone. Swoop back around and curve along the jawline. Think of this application as creating a number-3 shape.

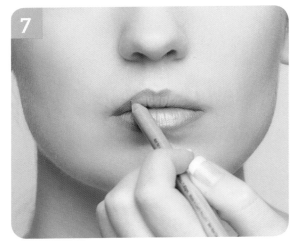

7

Line the lips with apricot lip pencil.

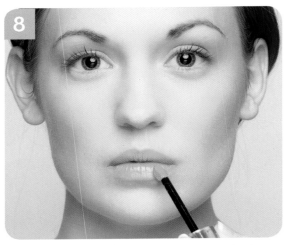

8

Apply apricot lip gloss to accentuate the lips.

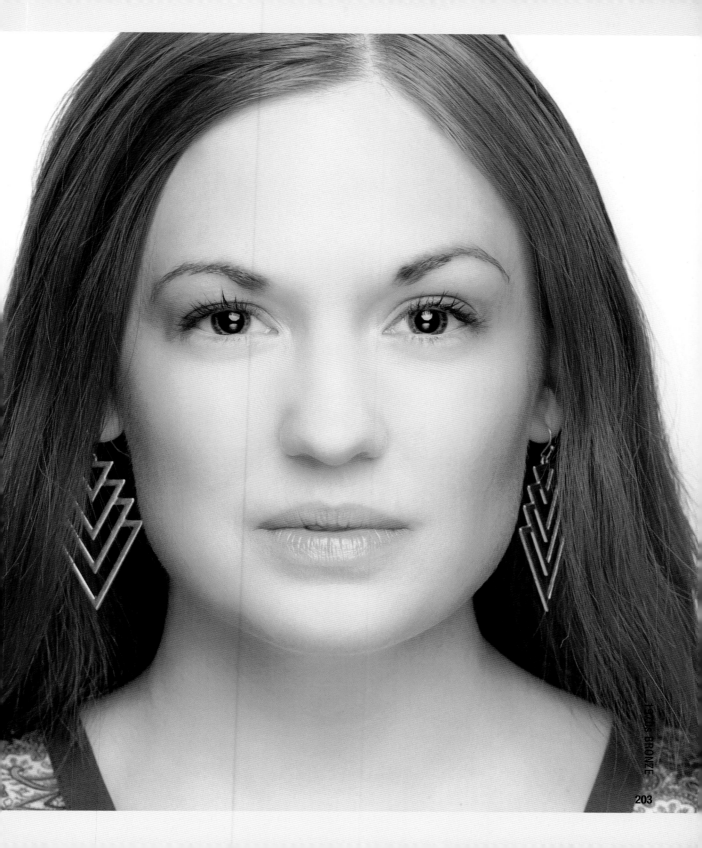

METALLIC
smoky eye

The typical smoky eye is created by blending grays and blacks onto the eyelid. This look uses a metallic silver shadow in place of the gray, giving a contemporary twist to the traditional smoky eye. Metallic looks like this are especially fabulous for dark skin tones.

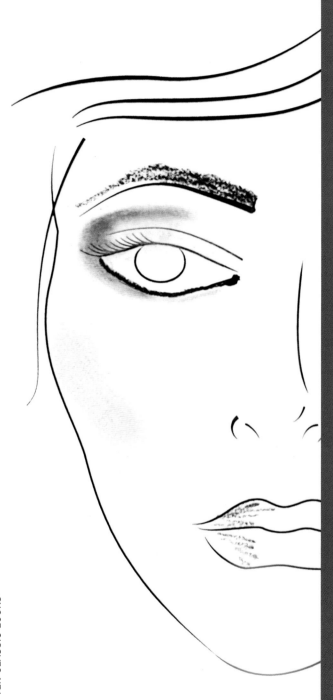

METALLIC SMOKY EYE
FACE SHEET

FOUNDATION/CONCEALER:
Orange-brown cream primer
Full-coverage liquid foundation

CORRECTIVE MAKEUP:
Cream highlight
Brown cream contour
Tinted setting powder

EYES:
Black eyeliner pencil
Highlight cream eye shadow
White eye shadow
Gunmetal metallic eye shadow
Black eye shadow
Silver metallic liquid eye
shadow
Black mascara

CHEEKS:
Orange cream blush

LIPS:
Flesh-colored lip pencil
Apricot lip gloss

METALLIC SMOKY EYE
PROFILE SHEET

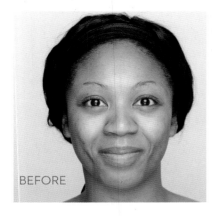

BEFORE

NAME:	Ashley
AGE:	32
FACE SHAPE:	diamond
EYE SHAPE:	wide set and monolid
EYE COLOR:	brown
EYEBROWS:	soft angled
NOSE:	wide
LIPS:	wide
SKIN TYPE:	combination
AREAS OF CONCERN:	dark spots
SKIN TONE:	cool
PRIMER:	orange
FOUNDATION:	liquid

Tools

Medium eye shadow brush

Concealer brush

Disposable latex sponge

Powder brush

Large eye shadow brush

Angle brush

Dual-fiber brush

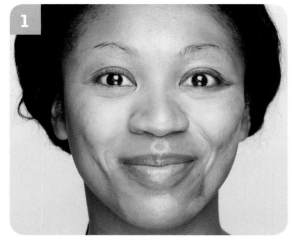

Apply orange-brown cream primer under the eyes and brow bones, around the nose, on the chin, and on any other trouble spots.

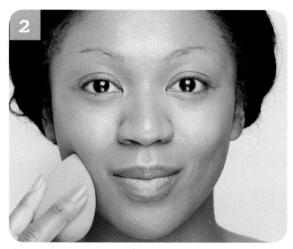

Apply full-coverage liquid foundation.

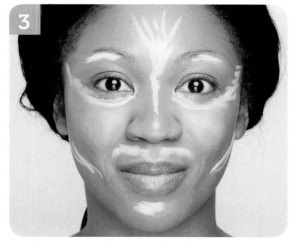

Apply cream highlight under the brow bones, between the eyebrows, and up the forehead. Continue application down the center of the nose, under the eyelids to the hairline, above the lips, under the hollows of the cheeks, and on the middle of the chin.

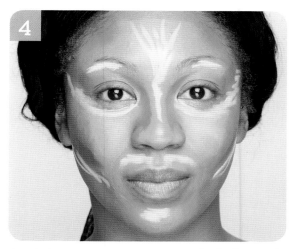

Apply brown cream contour to the hollows of the cheeks, under the chin, above the highlight in the temple, and from along the sides of nose to the corners of eyes.

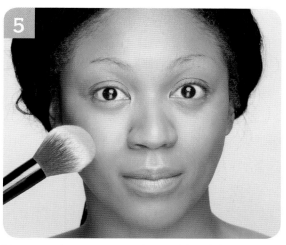

Use tinted setting powder to blend the contour.

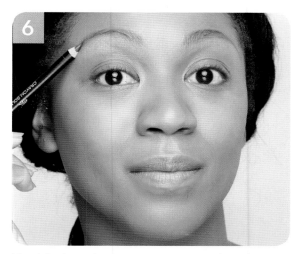

Use black eyeliner to create curved eyebrows.

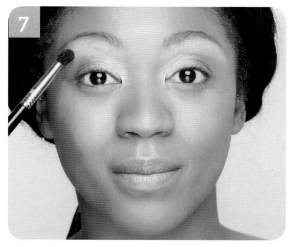

Apply highlight cream eye shadow to the brow bones and white eye shadow in the center of your nose contour. Continue by placing white eye shadow in the corners of the eyes and brushing it up and into the brow bones.

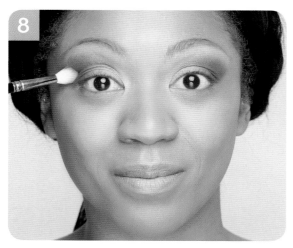

Apply gunmetal metallic eye shadow for contour in the crease, making sure to blend it into the outer edges of the lids.

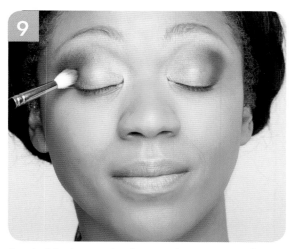

Apply black eye shadow to the corners of each eye and blend to the crease, making sure to blend in circular motions. This creates the smoky-eye effect.

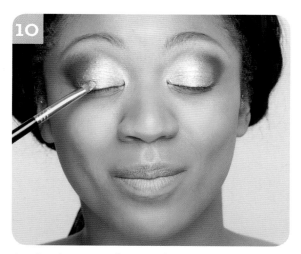

Apply silver metallic eye shadow to the lower lids.

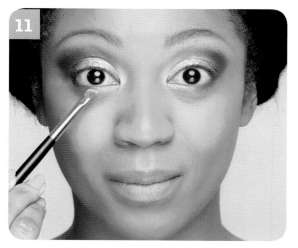

Using black eye shadow, create a soft, smoky line starting on the outside corner of the lower lash line and moving to the middle of the lower lash line. Brush slowly back and forth to blend. Apply silver metallic eye shadow from the tear duct to the middle of the lower lid, connecting it to the black shadow. Swipe back and forth to diffuse and blend the colors.

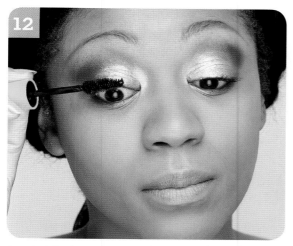

Apply black eyeliner in the water line of each eye. Finish the eyes by applying black mascara.

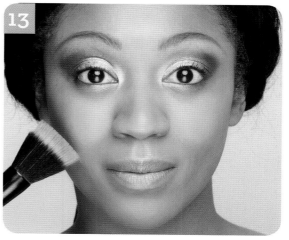

Apply orange blush to the apples of the cheeks.

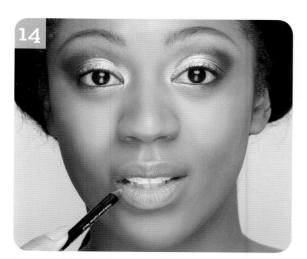

Line and fill the lips with flesh-colored lip pencil.

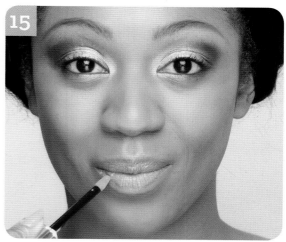

Finish the lip by applying apricot lip gloss.

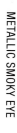

METALLIC SMOKY EYE

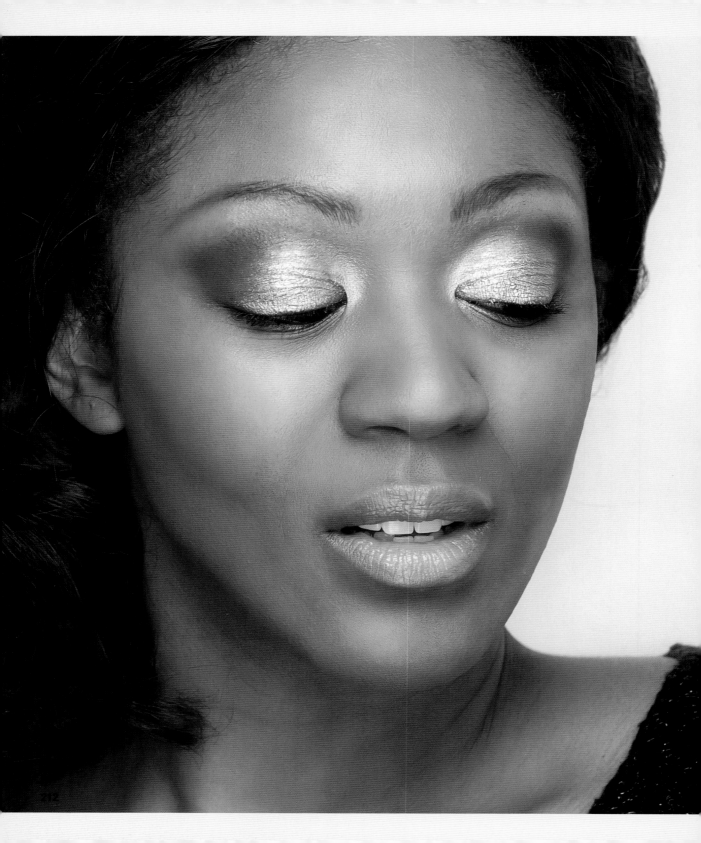

Cheek Color for Cool Tones

Because Ashley has cool, bluish tones, orange blush neutralizes to a more natural color, resulting in warmth.

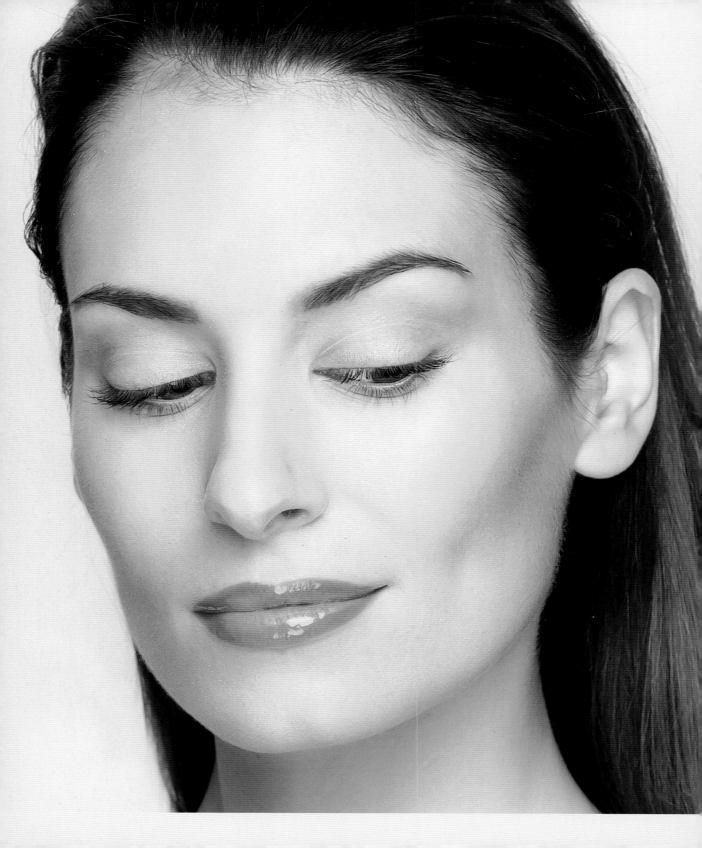

all about the
LIPS

It seems so easy to focus on the eyes when creating a makeup look. However, don't underestimate the lips! There are so many gorgeous lip shades out there to play with—pinks, reds, and even deep oranges can be stunning. The goal in a focused lip look is to keep the makeup natural; very little eyelid color and light foundation are all you need to set your lips up for success. Once you're done, you can throw on a big pair of sunglasses and be ready for a day of shopping!

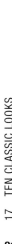

ALL ABOUT THE LIPS
FACE SHEET

FOUNDATION/CONCEALER:
Liquid foundation

CORRECTIVE MAKEUP:
None

EYES:
Ivory eye shadow
Matte taupe eye shadow
Black mascara

CHEEKS:
Peach blush

LIPS:
Lip exfoliant
Lip balm
Pink-orange lip pencil
Pink-orange lipstick
Pale gold shimmer lip gloss

ALL ABOUT THE LIPS
PROFILE SHEET

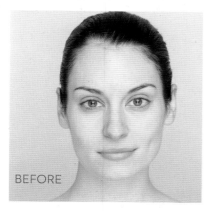

BEFORE

NAME: Erin

AGE: 26

FACE SHAPE: oblong (rectangle)

EYE SHAPE: upturned

EYE COLOR: blue

EYEBROWS: soft angled

NOSE: natural

LIPS: wide

SKIN TYPE: normal

AREAS OF CONCERN: none

SKIN TONE: cool

PRIMER: none

FOUNDATION: liquid

Tools

Disposable latex sponge

Cotton swab

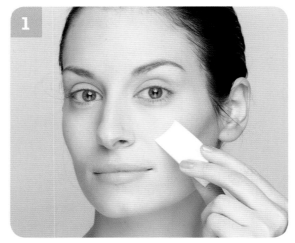

Apply matte liquid foundation all over the face.

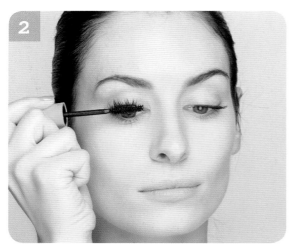

Apply ivory eye shadow all over each eyelid, starting at the brow bone and working your way down. Apply matte taupe eye shadow in each crease. Apply black mascara.

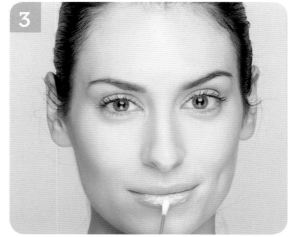

Apply peach blush to the cheeks, making sure to follow the natural cheekbones. Place lip exfoliant on a cotton swab and gently rub back and forth over the lips to remove dead skin.

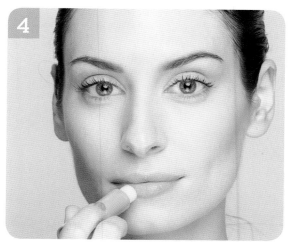

Apply lip balm to rehydrate the lips and provide a healthy surface for the lip color.

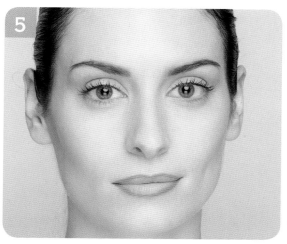

Apply pink-orange lip pencil along the natural lip line.

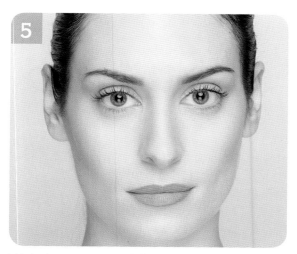

With the same pencil, fill in the lips.

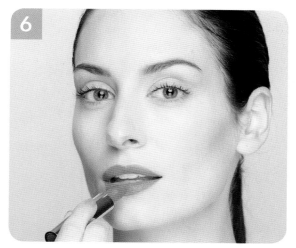

Apply pink-orange lipstick.

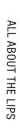

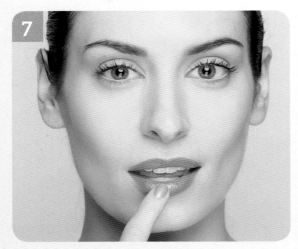

To create depth on the lips, apply pale gold shimmer lip gloss in the center of the upper and bottom lips.

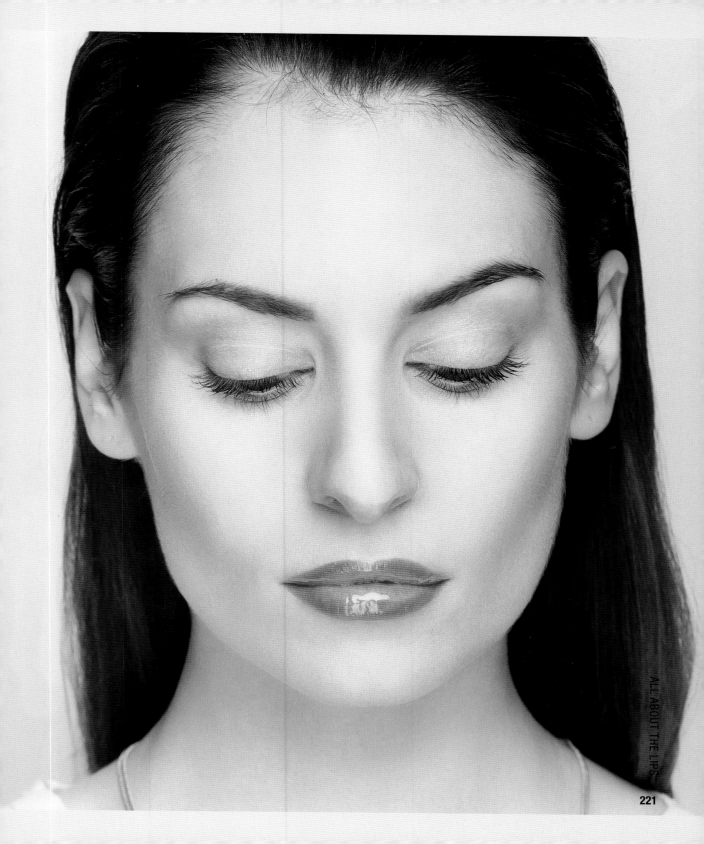

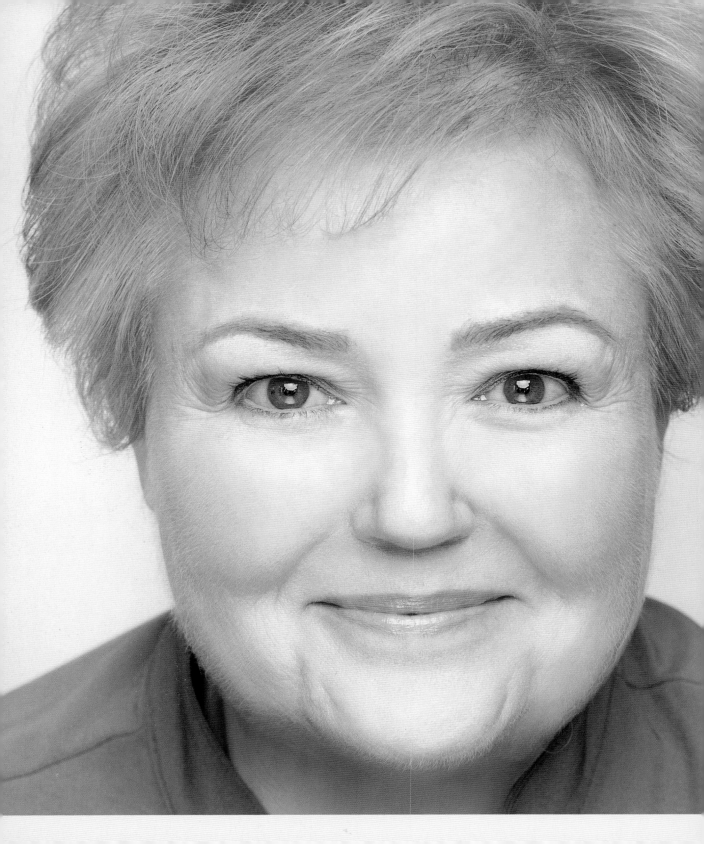

MATURE
mineral

Mineral makeup is a great choice for any skin type, but it is especially beneficial to mature skin. Mineral is lightweight, allowing the skin to breathe, plus it has light-diffusing properties that soften the appearance of lines and wrinkles. Finally, minerals don't settle into lines and wrinkles the way traditional liquid foundations and powders might. Unlike traditional makeup, this tutorial should leave mature skin looking fresh and dewy.

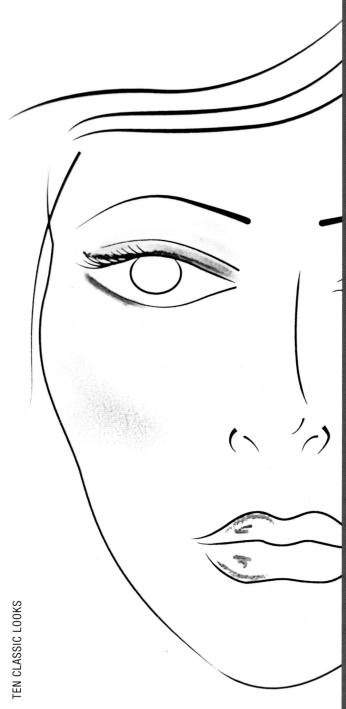

MATURE
MINERAL
FACE SHEET

FOUNDATION/CONCEALER:
Mineral cream concealer (one shade lighter)
Golden light mineral foundation
Hydrating mist

EYES:
Light brown eye shadow
Warm honey mineral foundation contour
Vanilla mineral eye shadow
Warm taupe mineral eye shadow
Dark brown shimmer eye shadow
Medium brown eyeliner
Black mascara

CHEEKS:
Pink-orange mineral blush

LIPS:
Nude lip pencil
Flesh-colored tinted lip gloss

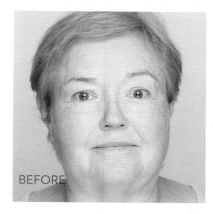

BEFORE

MATURE MINERAL
PROFILE SHEET

NAME: Camille

AGE: 61

FACE SHAPE: square

EYE SHAPE: hooded

EYE COLOR: green

EYEBROWS: curved

NOSE: thin

LIPS: combination

SKIN TYPE: sensitive

AREAS OF CONCERN: none

SKIN TONE: warm

PRIMER: none

FOUNDATION: mineral

Tools

Concealer brush

Kabuki brush

Angle brush

Large eye shadow brush

Medium eye shadow brush

Cotton swab

Blush brush

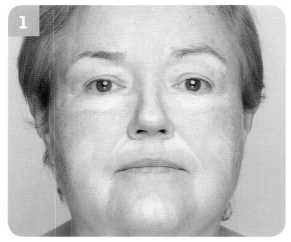

Apply concealer one shade lighter than your skin tone under the brow bones, from the corners of the eyes to underneath the eyes, on the bridge and around the nose, on the chin, and anywhere you need to diminish redness.

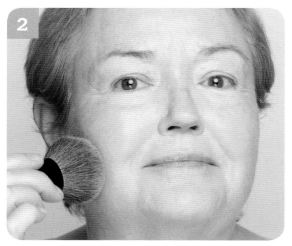

Buff golden light mineral foundation into the skin all over.

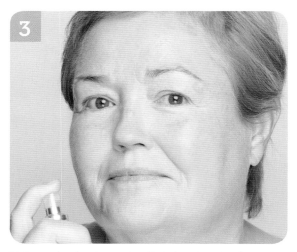

Using a hydrating mist, lightly mist the face to give an airbrushed feel and look.

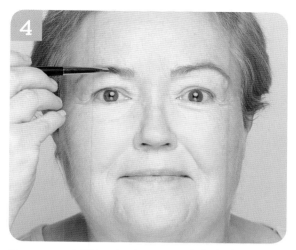

Groom and fill in the brows with light brown eye shadow.

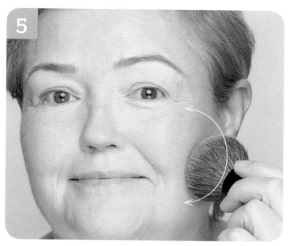

Use warm honey mineral foundation within the contours of the cheeks, applying it in a C shape toward the jawline.

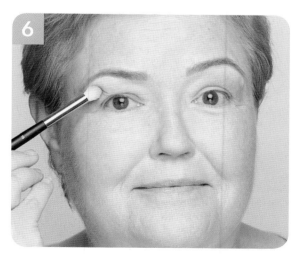

Apply vanilla mineral eye shadow to each eye starting under the brow bone and working it over the lid. Next, apply warm taupe mineral eye shadow in a U shape, angling it on the outside of the eyelid and down the corner of the eyelid to create a crease.

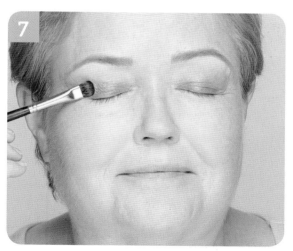

Apply dark brown shimmer eye shadow in a half-moon shape to create dimension and depth for the eyes.

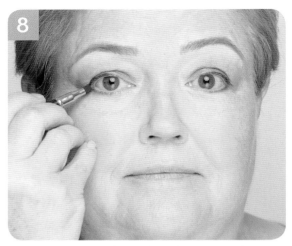

For each eye, apply medium brown eyeliner on the outer half of the bottom lash line. Using a cotton swab, gently blend the liner back and forth to smudge the line.

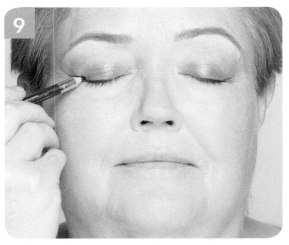

Apply medium brown eyeliner on the outside corners of the upper lash lines, gently swooping upward at the end to give the eyes a lift. Apply more eyeliner from the middle of the eyes to the tear ducts and smudge lightly.

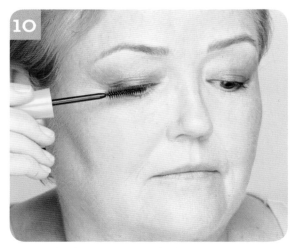

Apply black mascara on the lashes to make them pop. (For a softer look, use brown mascara instead.)

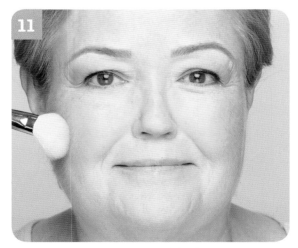

Brush pink-orange mineral blush on the cheeks and into the apples of the cheeks.

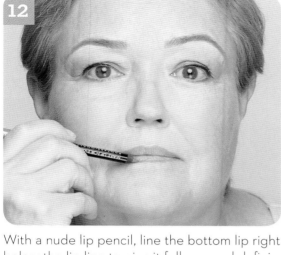

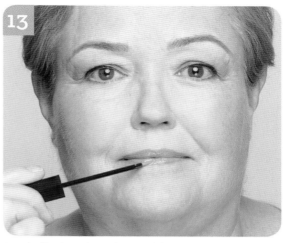

With a nude lip pencil, line the bottom lip right below the lip line to give it fullness and definition. Fill in the lips.

Apply flesh-colored tinted lip gloss to give a little shimmer to the lips.

Mature Makeup Tips

With mature skin, you want to stay as minimalistic and natural as possible when it comes to your makeup application, helping to create a sophisticated, classic look. Avoid matte foundation bases, as these will only enhance dry patches of skin. Also, don't use powders to set your base, as those will end up sitting in lines and creases. Creams, gels, and liquids all work well on mature skin because they will create a dewy fresh finish that won't settle into lines like powder does.

Mature Skin Application Note

If you have a heavy eyelid, don't lift the skin of the eye to apply eye shadow. Mature skin lacks elasticity, so the eye shadow placement will be incorrect. Instead, apply eye shadow to the visible part of the eyelid.

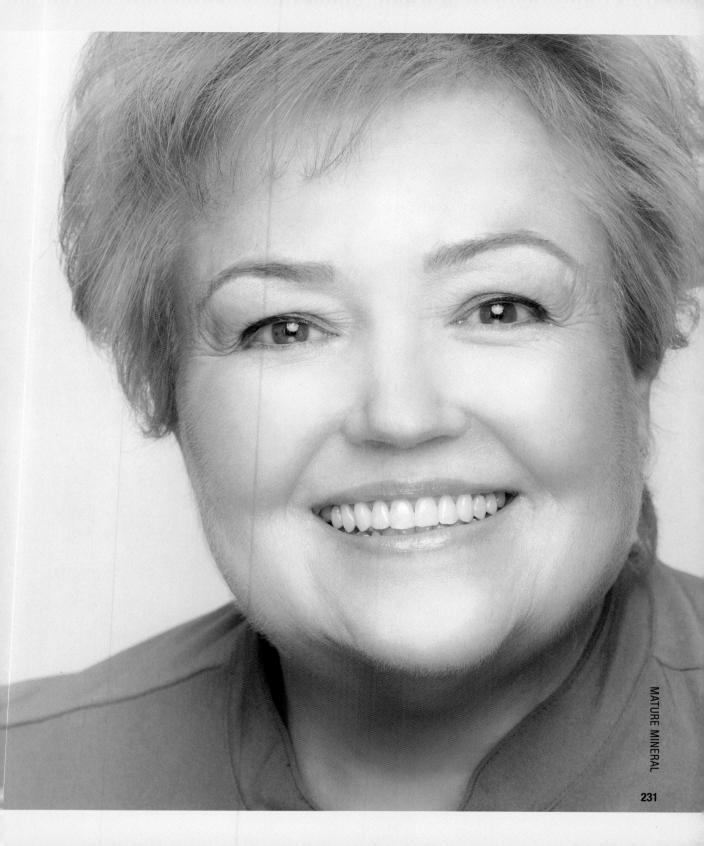

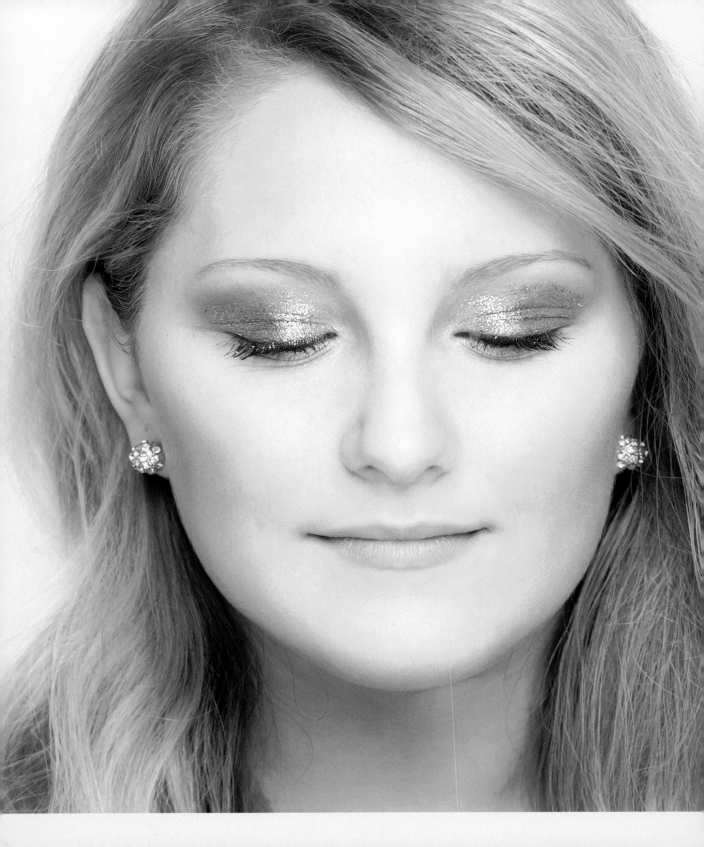

youthful GLITTER

Cosmetic glitter is a great makeup tool for creating a fun and sassy look. It is nontoxic and comes in many different fun shades. While this strong of a glitter look should be left to the very young, older women can certainly include elements for an evening look. Because glitter should be the leading player in this youthful look, keep your cheeks and lips neutral!

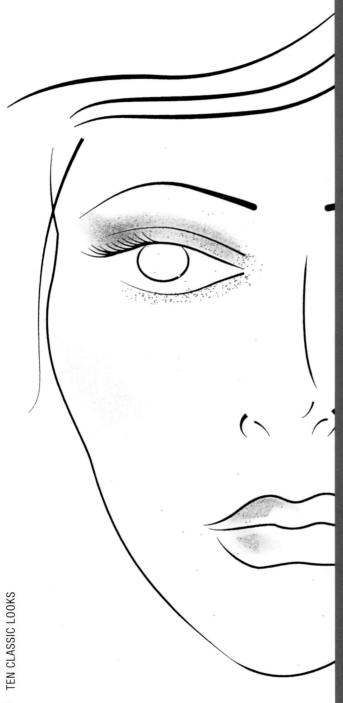

YOUTHFUL GLITTER
FACE SHEET

FOUNDATION/CONCEALER:
Cream concealer
Moisture tint foundation

CORRECTIVE MAKEUP:
Powder highlight

EYES:
Taupe eye shadow
Emerald green shimmer eye shadow
Frosty white eye shadow
Black mascara
Jade green cosmetic glitter

CHEEKS:
Dusty rose powder blush

LIPS:
Fleshy pink matte lip pencil

YOUTHFUL GLITTER
PROFILE SHEET

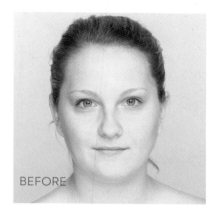

BEFORE

NAME:	Brooke
AGE:	19
FACE SHAPE:	square
EYE SHAPE:	downturned
EYE COLOR:	blue-green
EYEBROWS:	curved
NOSE:	thin
LIPS:	combination
SKIN TYPE:	dry
AREAS OF CONCERN:	none
SKIN TONE:	cool
PRIMER:	none
FOUNDATION:	liquid

Tools

Blush brush

Angle brush

Large eye shadow brush

Medium eye shadow brush

Cotton swab

Tissues

Cosmetic glue (optional)

Scotch tape

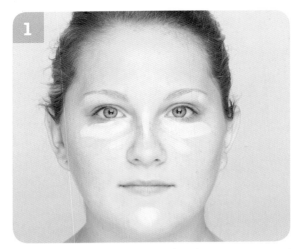

Apply cream concealer under the eyes, around the nose, and on the chin.

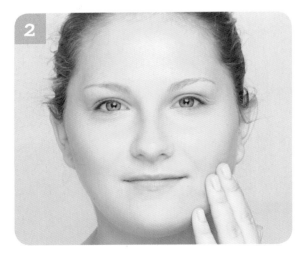

Apply moisture tint foundation all over the face.

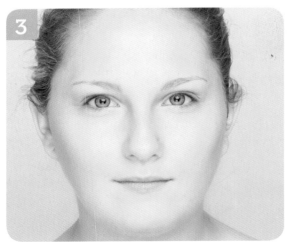

Apply powder highlight on the brow bones, cheekbones, and nose.

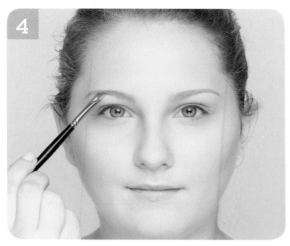

Apply taupe eye shadow to the eyebrows to reshape them.

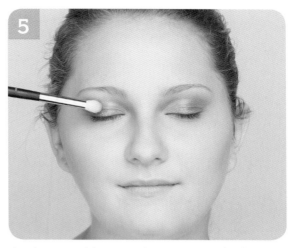

Apply emerald green shimmer eye shadow on the lid up to just above the crease. This creates a background color to the glitter, particularly for hooded eyes.

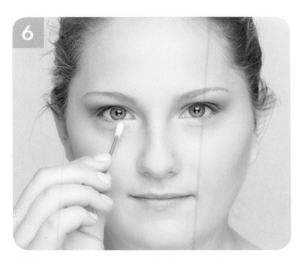

With a cotton swab, apply frosty white eye shadow in the corners of the eye and lightly under the bottom lash line.

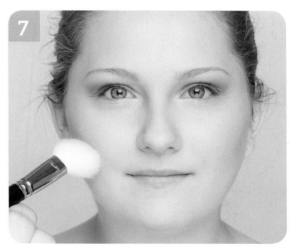

Brush on dusty rose blush, blending it into the apples of the cheek.

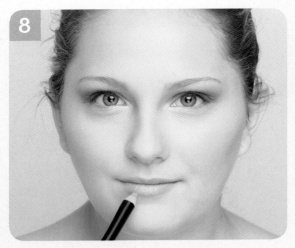

Apply fleshy pink matte lip pencil right above the natural lip line to create fuller lips.

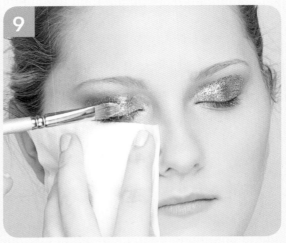

For each eye, place a tissue under the eyelash, close the eye, and gently press jade green cosmetic glitter on the eyelid with a brush. Cosmetic glitter glue can be used if necessary to secure the glitter.

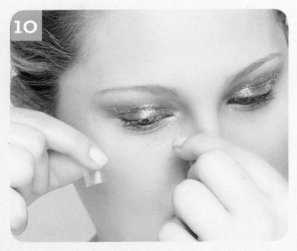

Use a piece of Scotch tape to remove any glitter that has fallen onto the cheeks or anywhere else on the face. Apply several coats of black mascara.

Glitter Warning

When using cosmetic glitter, less is more. It is easy to make the glitter look messy by applying too much.

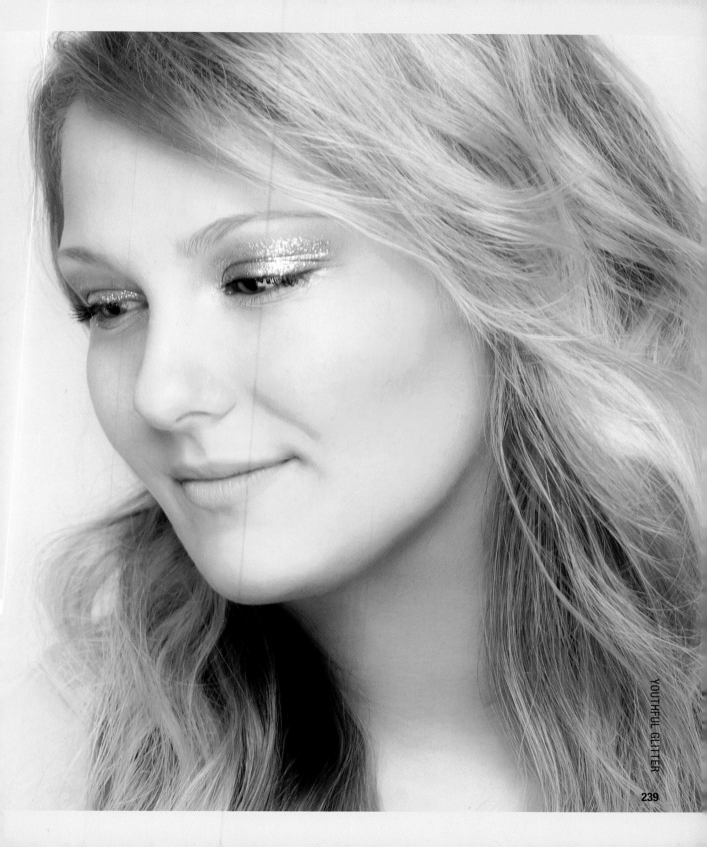

PART 4
APPENDIX

GLOSSARY

airbrushing   A combination of a concentrated pigment with a flow of air. It essentially mists the makeup onto your skin, creating a natural silkscreen effect.

beauty sponge   A sponge applicator without edges. You can use a beauty sponge to blend makeup after applying it with your fingers or a makeup brush.

bridge   The cartilage running down the center of the nose.

bronzer   A product used to imitate a natural suntan. It is considered a natural look and is often used for everyday wear. It highlights your cheekbones and contours your face. Bronzer is an easy way to enhance color and provide shimmer to your skin tone.

chemical exfoliant   A product that utilizes chemicals such as hydroxy acids (lactic acid, salicylic acid, and glycolic acid), retinol (vitamin A), and enzymes (Papain, Bromelain, and protease enzymes from *Bacillus* microbes) to create cell turnover in the epidermis. This stimulates the formation of normal, healthy skin.

complementary colors   Colors that are opposite each other on the color wheel. When combined in the right proportions, they create white or black. Complementary colors can help you choose which shades work best for everything from your skin's undertone to your eyes, lips, and nails.

concealer   A flesh-toned cosmetic product used to cover dark circles, discoloration, age spots, and blemishes. It is similar to foundation, but thicker.

contour   Giving shape to an area of your face and enhancing your facial structure through the use of makeup. Contour uses a powder or cream makeup product typically one to two shades darker than your skin color.

corrective makeup   Using highlight (light) and contour (dark/shadow) to change the shape of your face. Corrective makeup highlights features you find attractive and hides your less flattering features.

emphasis   The areas to which you want to draw attention. Makeup uses color as emphasis to direct attention to different parts of your face, such as your lips or your eyes.

exfoliant   Products designed to remove dead cells from the surface of your skin. *See also* mechanical exfoliant *and* chemical exfoliant.

eyelash curler   A tool used to curl your eyelashes prior to applying mascara or false eyelashes.

eyelash primer   A cosmetic that coats your eyelashes, protecting them from damage from mascara. Primers provide moisture to dry lashes and allow your mascara to go on evenly.

face sheet   A document used to record what cosmetics you used to achieve a certain look and where you placed those products on your face. A face sheet is typically broken into three sections: eyes, cheeks, and lips.

ferrule   Pronounced like *feral*, the metal portion of a makeup brush that holds the bristles in place.

foundation   Skin-colored makeup used to cover and even your skin tone, cover flaws, and sometimes change the color of your face.

highlight   The process of lightening an area to bring it forward or make it more prominent. Highlight uses powder or cream makeup products one to shades lighter than your skin color.

kabuki brush   A brush specially made for the application of mineral makeup. The design of the brush—a short handle and dense bristles—assists in a heavier application necessary for this makeup.

mechanical exfoliant   A product that employs the use of either a tool (for example, a brush or sponge) or substrate (for example, corn cob meal, rice bran, date seed powder, or oatmeal) to stimulate cell turnover. Depending on the amount of friction and nature of abrasive used, a mechanical exfoliant loosens and reduces the outer layer of skin.

mineral makeup   A makeup that contains 100 percent minerals (such as titanium dioxide, zinc oxide, mica, and iron oxide) and is free of organic dyes, preservatives, and fragrance. Many ancient cultures used ground-up natural minerals as a means of applying color to the skin for decoration, camouflage, and war paint.

monolid   An eye shape in which you have little to no crease in your eye and no brow bone. With a monolid, there is a fairly flat surface between your eyelid and your eyebrow.

pH   A measurement of the acidity or alkalinity of a solution. The pH of healthy skin is 4.5 to 5.5.

primary colors   Refers to a group of colors that can be mixed together to make all other colors. Red, yellow, and blue are primary colors.

primer   A cream or lotion applied to improve the coverage and duration of your makeup. A primer is applied before a concealer. *See also* tinted primer.

salicylic acid   A beta-hydroxy acid used to treat acne.

secondary colors   A combination of two or more primary colors. Orange, green, and violet are secondary colors.

setting powder   A type of powder used for reducing sweat on your face, setting cream foundation, and blending your contour.

shimmer   A type of eye shadow that has light-reflecting materials included. Shimmer gives depth and interest to the many eye shadow shades available.

smoky eye   A dramatic style of eye makeup that gives your eyes a dark, smoky appearance. Its popularity began in the 1920s. The typical smoky eye uses black and gray eye shadows and black liner applied in a circular pattern around the eyes.

SPF   The acronym for sun protection factor, refers to the ability of a sunscreen to block ultraviolet rays, which cause sunburns. SPF is added to many moisturizers and foundations so your skin is protected.

T-zone   Where your skin tends to become the most oily. To find your T-zone, draw an imaginary line across your forehead and another line from your nose to your chin.

tattoo cover   A very thick cosmetic product with a matte finish that's used to cover up the dark and multi-colored ink of a tattoo.

tertiary colors   A combination of a primary and secondary color. Red-orange, red-violet, yellow-orange, yellow-green, blue-violet, and blue-green are tertiary colors.

tinted primer   A cream or lotion available in red, green, yellow, or violet. It is used to neutralize problem areas on the skin, such as rosacea, acne, dark circles, and any other skin discolorations.

toner   A skin care product that's balanced to return skin to its proper pH. Additionally, toners remove excess debris and reduce pore size.

UV rays   Refers to ultraviolet radiation, or the amount of energy radiating from the sun. Products like sunscreen, moisturizers, and foundations include a sun protection factor to protect your skin from these harmful rays.

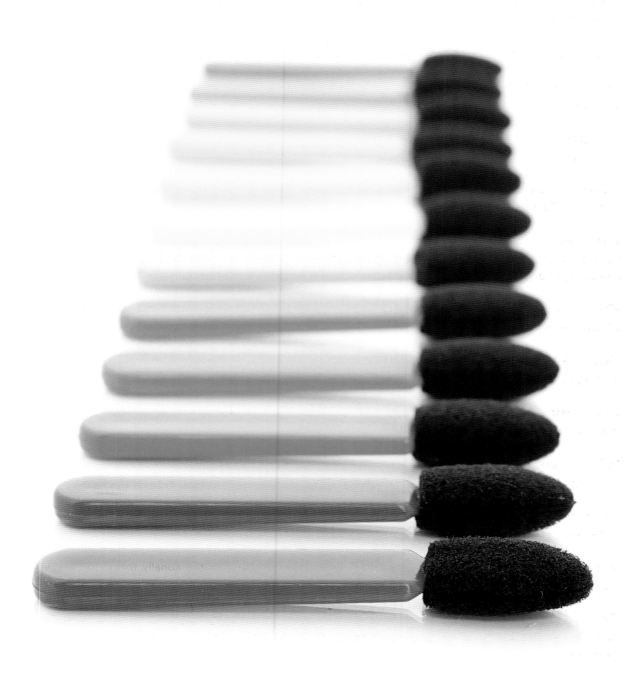

INDEX

1940s style, 181–187
1950s style, 189–195
1970s style, 197–203

A

acids, toners, 27
acne, cleansers, 25
almond eyes, 115
angle brush, 9
    contouring, 75

B

baby wipes, 13
blending brush, 11
blush. See also cheek color
    face shape and, 68–71
blush brush, 8
bridge of the nose, 74
bronzer, 65
    brush, 10
    contouring and, 39
brow brush, 12
brushes
    angle brush, 9
    blending, 11
    blush, 8
    bronzer, 10
    brows, 12
    cleaner, 17
    concealer, 10

density, 7
dual-fiber, 10
eye shadow, 9, 11
eyeliner, 11
fan, 12
ferrule, 7
fibers, 6–7
foundation, 10, 50
handle, 7
kabuki, 10
lips, 10
mineral makeup, 47
powder, 8, 83
shapes, 7
smudge, 11

C

camouflage cover, 60–61
cheek color, 64
    application tips, 71
    bronzer, 65
    contouring, 66–67
    cream, 65
    face shape, 68–71
    highlighting, 66–67
    mineral, 65
    powder, 65
chemical exfoliants, 26
cleanser, 25
    brush cleaner, 17
    makeup remover, 16
close-set eyes, 116

colors
    eye shadow selection, 102
    foundation, 48
    lips, 137
    mascara, 123
    primer and, 54–55
    skin tone, 44–45
combination skin, 23
    moisturizer, 29
concave face profile, 35
concealer
    applying, 58
    brush, 10
    color-correcting, 57
    compact/container, 57
    cream, 56
    liquid, 56
    pencil, 57
    powder, 56
    redness, 58
    stick, 57
    tattoos, 60–61
    tinted moisturizer and, 49
    tube, 57
contouring
    cheeks, 66–67
    face shape and, 40–41, 68–71
    nose, 75–79
    powder blending, 85
    products, 38
convex face profile, 35
cool skin tone, 44
corrective makeup
    concealer, 57
    contouring, 38

eye shape, 115–119
    face profile, 35
    face segments, 34
    highlighter, 38
    shape of face, 36–37
    width of face, 36
cotton swabs, 13
creams
    cheek color, 65
    eye shadow, 100
    foundation, 46
    makeup, contouring and, 39
curling mascara, 122

D

deep-set eyes, 116
dewy finish, 49
diamond-shaped face, 37
    blush, 71
    contouring and, 41, 71
    highlighting, 71
disposable tools, 13
    lifespan, 18
disposing of makeup, 19
downturned eyes, 119
dry skin, 22
    moisturizer, 29
dual-fiber brush, 10

E

exfoliants, 26
expiration date of makeup, 19
eye creams, 28
eye shadow
    application, 104–105
    brushes, 9, 11

color selection, 102
    contouring and, 39
    cream, 100
    eye color and, 103
    eyebrow fill in, 94
    as eyeliner, 108
    glitter, 101
    loose powder, 100
    matte, 101
    metallic, 101
    mineral, 100
    pressed powder, 100
    sheer, 101
    shimmer, 101
eye shape, correcting, 115
eyebrows
    angled, 89
    curved, 89
    face shape, 90–91
    filling in, 94–95
    flat, 89
    overtweezed, 88
    pencil, 94
    round, 89
    shaping, 88
    soft angled, 89
    stencil, 96
    threading, 92
    tweezing, 92
    waxing, 92–93
eyelashes
    curler, 126
    extensions, 130–131
    false, 127–129
    mascara, 122–125
    strips, 128–129
eyeliner
    application, 109
    brush, 11
    by era, 110–111

    eye shadow, 108
    gel pot, 108
    liquid, 108
    pencil, 108
eyes
    almond shaped, 115
    brow bone, 114
    close-set, 116
    crease, 114
    dark circles, 28, 58
    deep-set, 116
    downturned, 119
    eyelid, 114
    fine lines, 28
    hooded, 118
    lash lines, 114
    monolid, 118
    prominent, 117
    puffiness, 28
    small, 117
    tear ducts, 114
    upturned, 119
    wide set, 115
    wrinkles, 28

F–G

face profile, 35
face segments, 34
face shape, 36–37
    blush, 68–71
    contouring, 40–41, 68–71
    eyebrows, 90–91
    highlighting, 40–41, 68–71
face sheet, 148–149
false eyelashes, strips, 128–129
fan brush, 12
fingers for foundation application,
   50

food for good skin, 25
foundation
    applying, 51
    brush, 10
    coverage, 48
    cream, 46
    finishes, 49
    full coverage, 48
    liquid, 46
    mineral makeup, 47
    pressed powder, 46
    testing, 48
    tinted, 46
    tools, 50

gel pot eyeliner, 108
glitter, makeup style, 223–239

H–I–J

heart-shaped face, 37
    blush, 70
    contouring and, 41, 70
    highlighting, 70
highlighter, 38
    cheeks, 66–67
    face shape and, 40–41, 68–71
    nose, 75–79
    powder blending, 85
hooded eyes, 118
hydrating mist, 85

K–L

kabuki brush, 10, 83
    mineral makeup, 47

lash-defining mascara, 122
lengthening mascara, 122
lip balm, 135

lip brush, 10
lip color, 137
    balancing lip shape, 139–140
lip gloss, 135
lip liner, 138
lip pencil, 134
    lining lips, 138
lip stain, 135
lips
    lining, 138
    style focus, 215–221
lipstick, 134
    palette, creating, 136
    setting, 135
    stains on glasses, 140
liquid eyeliner, 108
liquid foundation, 46
liquid skin as tattoo cover, 61
loose powder, 82

M

makeup
    disposing of, 19
    eyes and, 114
makeup looks
    dramatic evening, 171–179
    elegant evening, 161–169
makeup remover, 16
makeup sponges, 13
    contouring, 75
makeup styles
    1940s, 181–187
    1950s, 189–195
    1970s, 197–203
    daytime natural, 153–159
    glitter, 233–239
    mature, 223–231
    metallic style with smoky eye,
      205–213

mascara
    application, 125
    clumps, 125
    color, 123
    curling, 122
    lash-defining, 122
    lengthening, 122
    primer, 122
    smudge-proof, 122
    volumizing, 122
    wand types, 13, 124
    waterproof, 122
matte finish, 49
mature skin
    makeup style, 223–231
    moisturizer, 29
mechanical exfoliants, 26
medium coverage foundation, 48
metallic style with smoky eye,
    205–213
mineral makeup, 47
    cheek color, 65
    eye shadow, 100
    mature skin, 223–231
    powder, 82
moisturizers, 29
    tinted moisturizer, 46, 49
monolid eyes, 118

N

neutral skin tone, 45
normal skin, 22
    moisturizer, 29
nose
    contouring, 75–79
    highlighting, 75–79
    parts, 74
nostrils, 74

O

oblong-shaped face, 37
  blush, 70
  contouring and, 41, 70
  highlighting, 70
oil-based makeup remover, 17
oily skin, 22
  moisturizer, 29
oval-shaped face, 36
  blush, 68
  contouring and, 40, 68
  highlighting, 68

P

pencil eyeliner, 108
pH balance, 27
powder
  basic, 84
  brush, 8
  cheek color, 65
  contouring and, 39
  eye shadow, 100
  highlight/contour blending, 85
  loose, 82
  mineral, 82
  pressed, 82
  pressed powder foundation, 46
  tinted, 82
  tools, 83
  translucent, 82
primer, 54–55
primer mascara, 122
profile sheet, 147
prominent eyes, 117

Q–R

redness, concealer, 58
round-shaped face, 36
  blush, 69
  contouring and, 40, 69
  highlighting, 69

S

sanitation
  brush cleaner, 16
  disposable applicators, 18
  makeup remover, 16
  pencil sharpeners, 18
  pencils, 18
scrubs, 26
sensitive skin, 23
  moisturizer, 29
shape of face, 36–37
sheer to light coverage foundation, 48
shimmer finish, 49
sidewalls of the nose, 74
skin care, 21
  cleansers, 25
  exfoliants, 26
  eye creams, 28
  foods, 24
  moisturizers, 29
  skin types, 22–23
  toners, 27
skin tone, 44–45
  lip color, 137
  uneven, 58
skin types, 22–23
  moisturizers, 29
smudge brush, 11
smudge-proof mascara, 122

SPF

SPF (sun protection factor), 29
sponges, 13
  contouring, 75
  foundation, 50
square-shaped face, 36
  blush, 69
  contouring and, 40, 69
  highlighting, 69
stencil for eyebrows, 96
styles, lip focus, 215–221

T

tattoo covering, 60–61
thin lips, 140
threading eyebrows, 92
tinted moisturizer, 46
  creating your own, 49
tinted powder, 39, 82
tinted primer, 54–55
tip of the nose, 74
toners, 27
tools
  brushes, 6–12
  disposable, 13, 18
  eyebrow filling, 94
  foundation, 50
  in package, 5
  powder application, 83
translucent powder, 82
tweezing eyebrows, 92

U–V

upturned eyes, 119

vertical face profile, 35
volumizing mascara, 122

W–X–Y–Z

warm skin tone, 44
water-based makeup remover, 17
waterproof mascara, 122
waxing eyebrows, 92–93
wide lips, 139
wide-set eyes, 115
wrinkles, eyes, 28

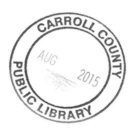